Enquiring into Healthcare Practice

First edition 1996

Published by
Macmillan Magazines Ltd
Porters South
4 Crinan Street
London N1 9XW

Companies and representatives throughout the world

Printed in Great Britain by
Grange Press
Southwick, West Sussex

ISBN 0 333 675290

CORE MEMBERS OF DEGREE TEAM

Cathy Hull, head of curriculum development and publishing, Macmillan Open Learning
Michelle Murtagh, editorial PA, Macmillan Open Learning
Elizabeth Redfern, education consultant (formerly assistant director for educational policy, English National Board)
Eimer Rogers, projects manager, Macmillan Open Learning
Simon Shaw, director, Cambridge Training and Development Ltd

DEGREE ADVISORY TEAM

Dai Hall, open and distance learning co-ordinator, Post Compulsory Education and Training, University of Greenwich
John Humphreys, head of school, Post Compulsory Education and Training, University of Greenwich
Debra Humphris, senior research fellow, Healthcare Evaluation Unit, St George's Hospital Medical School, London
Linda Husband, lecturer, Humberside College of Health and tutor/counsellor to Macmillan Open Learning DipHE students
Chris James, professor, University of Glamorgan Business School
Anne Palmer, education consultant to the University of Westminster
Richard Parish, director of school health and community studies, Sheffield Hallam University
Marianne Phillips, head of division, Macmillan Open Learning, and University Pathway Director for DipHE
Frank Quinn, director of healthcare education, Post Compulsory Education and Training, University of Greenwich
Gwilym Roberts, director of fieldwork studies, School of Occupational Therapy, London Hospital Medical College, University of London

MACMILLAN OPEN LEARNING ADVISORY COMMITTEE

Margaret Alexander, professor, Department of Nursing and Community Health, Glasgow Caledonian University
Sue Frost, director of adult and children's nursing, English National Board
Liz Gillies, professional officer, National Board for Nursing, Midwifery and Health Visiting for Scotland
Maureen Lavery, professional officer, National Board for Nursing, Midwifery and Health Visiting for Northern Ireland
Ann Ryall-Davies, director of professional services, Welsh National Board for Nursing, Midwifery and Health Visiting
Jeff Thompson, CBE, professor, School of Education, University of Bath

CRITICAL READERS FOR OVERALL DEGREE

Moya Davis, distance learning consultant and author
Anne Palmer, education consultant to the University of Westminster
Frank Quinn, director of healthcare education, Post Compulsory Education and Training, University of Greenwich
Gwilym Roberts, director of fieldwork studies, School of Occupational Therapy, London Hospital Medical College, University of London

CRITICAL READERS, ENQUIRING INTO HEALTHCARE PRACTICE UNIT

Isabel Bartram, head of school, School of Nursing and Midwifery, University of Wolverhampton, Walsall
Diana Coben, lecturer in continuing education/lifelong learning, Department of Education, Goldsmiths' College, University of London
Richard Edwards, senior lecturer, Institute of Educational Technology, Open University, Milton Keynes
Caroline Jarvis, professional education and development manager, St Richard's Hospital, The Royal West Sussex Trust, Chichester
Margaret Johnson, tutor, clinical education and practice, John Radcliffe Infirmary, Oxford
Martin Johnson, principal lecturer, School of Nursing Studies, University of Manchester
David Lewin, research and quality co-ordinator, Homerton School of Health Studies, Peterborough District Hospital
Di Marks-Maran, resource-based learning co-ordinator, Wolfson School of Health Sciences, Thames Valley University, London
Ken Martin, formerly lecturer in education, Goldsmiths' College, University of London and part-time tutor in psychology, Open University
Marlene Sinclair, tutor, Northern Area College of Nursing, Antrim Hospital site, Antrim, Northern Ireland
Claire Virgo, lecturer, City University School of Nursing and Midwifery, London

STUDENT TESTERS

Maggie Bean, Medical Chest Ward, Castle Hill Hospital, North Humberside
Natalie Christiansen, physiotherapy student, University of East London
Carol Edge, staff nurse, Ophthalmic Theatre, Victoria Hospital, Blackpool, Lancashire
Susanne Jupp, physiotherapy student, University of East London
Ellie Lindsay, district nursing sister, Allington NHS Trust, Ipswich
Helen Winterflood, Les Bourgs Hospice, St Andrews, Guernsey

EDITORIAL TEAM

Patsy Dale, chief sub-editor, Macmillan Open Learning
Pip Hardy, open learning editor
Cathy Lake, writer
Jenny Spouse, senior lecturer, School of Health Studies, Education Centre, Radcliffe Infirmary, Oxford
Gerard Tobin, senior lecturer/development co-ordinator, Oxford Clinical Eduational and Practice Team, John Radcliffe Hospital, Oxford

Special thanks to Sally Malin for her contribution to this unit

DESIGN

Clare Conway, designer, design studio, Macmillan Magazines
Graham Ogilvie, design studio manager, Macmillan Magazines
Steve Sullivan, graphic artist, Macmillan Magazines
Jane Walker, art director, Macmillan Magazines

PHOTOGRAPHS

Sue Lloyd, picture researcher, *Nursing Times*
Louise Thomas, picture researcher, *The Health Service Journal*

Special thanks to Medway NHS Trust for the use of their hospital as a photography resource

THE MACMILLAN OPEN LEARNING MISSION STATEMENT

The Macmillan Open Learning (MOL) programmes are based on the belief that the development of professional practice can be achieved only through the development of the professional as a person.

The MOL development team believe that:

- To become autonomous practitioners, professionals need to be self-directed, autonomous learners
- A programme of learning should focus on the learning process rather than the factual content
- The key to learning how to learn is through inquiry, reflection, evaluation and action
- An action-based, problem-solving approach to learning, combined with the reality of practice, will provide the appropriate stimulus and framework for learning.

Practice-based learning is the stimulus for raising standards of care generally within the learner's practice setting.

MOL programmes are therefore based on the following principles:

- A focus on learning rather than teaching
- Active involvement of learners, who have ownership of the learning, assessment and reflection processes
- Action-based, problem-solving approaches, which combine with the reality of practice to provide the stimulus and framework for learning
- Experiential approaches to learning which provide multiple and varied opportunities for learners to experience and/or act out the behaviours, knowledge and values of their own profession
- An emphasis on the integration of theory and practice in order that learners learn to structure concepts when thinking and making professional judgements in their practice.

Assessment is therefore integral to the learning process, rather than separate from it, and should:

- Enable and encourage learners to evaluate their own performance
- Focus on learners' critical analysis skills, and their ability to apply what has been learnt
- Enable and encourage learners to value personal theories and opinions.

Introduction
- ☐ You and the book
- ☐ Learning and reflection
- ☐ Assessment guidelines
- ☐ The personal profile
- ☐ Learning contracts
- ☐ Enquiring into practice

Section 1: What are you going to investigate?
- ☐ Introduction
- ☐ What does health care mean to you?
- ☐ The day-to-day reality
- ☐ Using the reflective process in enquiry
- ☐ Models of structured reflection — 1
- ☐ Models of structured reflection — 2
- ☐ Critical incident analysis
- ☐ Clarifying the question
- ☐ Analysing the concepts
- ☐ Recording your 'journey'
- ☐ Conclusion and References

Section 2: Methods of enquiry
- ☐ Introduction
- ☐ How do you find out things?
- ☐ Methods of enquiry used in health care
- ☐ What is enquiry?
- ☐ Enquiring into practice
- ☐ How useful is research?
- ☐ Quantitative and qualitative research
- ☐ Research paradigms — 1
- ☐ Research paradigms — 2
- ☐ Ways of knowing
- ☐ The issue of validity
- ☐ The language of research
- ☐ Terms commonly used in research
- ☐ Conclusion and References

Section 3: Exploring the literature
- ☐ Introduction
- ☐ Sources of information
- ☐ Starting a literature review
- ☐ An alternative approach
- ☐ Reading techniques
- ☐ Critical reading
- ☐ Recording a literature search
- ☐ Understanding statistical information
- ☐ Conclusion and References

Section 4: Planning and carrying out your enquiry
- ☐ Introduction
- ☐ Overview of the enquiry process
- ☐ Getting the scale right
- ☐ Managing your project
- ☐ More planning tools
- ☐ Stating the problem
- ☐ Organising a literature review
- ☐ Designing the study
- ☐ Samples
- ☐ Gathering data — 1
- ☐ Gathering data — 2
- ☐ Ethical issues
- ☐ Piloting and practising
- ☐ Data analysis for quantitative research
- ☐ Data analysis for qualitative research — 1
- ☐ Data analysis for qualitative research — 2
- ☐ Results, interpretation, conclusions and recommendations
- ☐ Limitations
- ☐ Conclusion and References

Section 5: Writing up your project
- ☐ Introduction
- ☐ How to present a research report
- ☐ Managing the writing process
- ☐ How to present a literature review
- ☐ Where do you go from here?
- ☐ Conclusion and References

You and the book

This book contains the supporting material for the core unit of the BSc (Hons) Professional Practice in Health Care. It offers an introduction to critical thinking, enquiry, analysis and research skills and will guide you through your work on the enquiry-based project.

The book presents a holistic and integrated approach to enquiry and will encourage you to use theoretical concepts to help you plan your independent enquiry. There are plenty of opportunities for testing out new skills and theories through your own experience and practice.

The option units in the degree programme may provide ideas for research and enquiry and can feed into the work you do on this unit just as your work on this unit will support what you do in the option units. The option units are shown in the box on the opposite page.

If you are undertaking the degree programme, you will be doing three option units as well as this core unit. You can study units separately, with support material in the form of a whole book (like this one) or as Professional Practice Study Units (PPSUs). Each PPSU contains one Section of a book. You can also buy a complete unit, with assessment, without having to register for a degree.

Studying PPSUs alone will enable you to develop some of the skills and capabilities you get from doing a degree. There are a number of advantages of studying several PPSUs:

- You will be able to study a topic in depth
- You will be able to appreciate the complexity of a topic from studying different approaches
- You will have the opportunity to synthesise knowledge from different sources
- By undertaking the assessment and the enquiry-based project you will have the opportunity to take the outcomes of a substantial, sustained piece of learning into practice.

For more information, contact:
Macmillan Open Learning
Porters South
Crinan Street
London N1 9XW

Students say: 'As I worked my way through the materials, I became more and more stimulated in my desire to put into practice what the material was encouraging me to understand.'

'. . . with this module I've found a "knowledgeable friend" to turn to for guidance and encouragement as I work through a research question – brilliant.'

'As I am now carrying out a research project whilst reading the material it was like a voice in my head reminding me of things to do or ensure a particular point was carried out correctly.'

The writer says: 'Whenever I get deeply involved in a subject, I start to make connections with other things I know about. All kinds of unexpected lights dawn and pennies drop, as knowledge and ideas from different areas of life come together. For me, this is one of the most exciting parts of writing. Normally, I keep these discoveries to myself, but in this project we were asked to share them with students. I hope the book that results is stimulating to read. It was certainly very stimulating to write.'

A critical reader says: 'The process of research is explored in such a way as to encourage the reader to engage in the 'doing' as well as making connections with their own experiences and practice settings.'

You may have had some ideas about what to expect in this unit. You may want to write them down, or draw a picture or diagram of your initial impression of the unit. If you do, your learning journal or reflective diary is a good place.

Your ideas may change as you work through the unit. Keep track of your thoughts and feelings by writing or drawing when you notice changes.

Taking charge

People learn in different ways, so use this book in a way that suits how you learn best. Some people like to start at the beginning and work through to the end. Others prefer a less systematic approach and like to take in different points of view as they go along. Links between Sections are built into the text, so you may find yourself going from one Section to another. There is no particular reason to read the various Sections in the order in which they are presented.

In general, it is more rewarding to decide for yourself how you will learn rather than have other people decide for you, and you can still achieve the assessment criteria if you are doing the degree (see pages 6-7).

Layout

The book has five Sections, with each Section divided into topics.

Most topics take up two facing pages – a double page spread. Read the book in this way – looking at both pages together as a whole. On most pages there is space for you to note your own views.

The top half of the page contains the kind of information which will stimulate you into researching and finding out more about the topic. The bottom half of the page has different sorts of information and gives you the opportunity to do something with it. There are activities, discussion points, quotes, references, charts, diagrams, current debates, case studies and ideas for assessment topics. However, you can read the bottom half of the page before the top half or mix them in any way that helps you to think and learn.

Boxes with dotted lines round them are Activity boxes, which contain material suggesting you do or think about some particular aspect relating to the text. Boxes that are tinted contain further references, quotes and comments.

Core Unit: Enquiring into Healthcare Practice

Healthcare Evaluation

Complementary Therapies and Healthcare Practice

Health Care and the Information Age

Health Promotion in Professional Practice

Influences in Health Care: Media perspectives

Professional Relationships: Influences on health care

Values and the Person: Ideas that influence health care

As you work on this unit, draw your own links with the option units you have chosen to study.

Learning and reflection

Reflective learning

When you are learning, it helps to reflect on the new ideas coming into your mind. You can do this by having a conversation with yourself, or with other people. But it is a particular sort of conversation: you will be asking questions, explaining, disagreeing, trying to get to the heart of the matter, turning things over in your mind, worrying about them. It could be useful to write some of this down, maybe in a learning journal or a reflective diary where you could be writing about:

- The process of learning
- The consequences of what has been learned
- What you discover about yourself as you learn.

Don't worry if things you read about in the book seem hazy for a time – that often happens when people are learning. Making notes and talking to others can help to clarify things and bring them into focus. Feed uncertainties into your writing and discussions, and into your personal profile as well (see pages 8-9).

Activities

When you come across an Activity, decide if you want to do it. You will be able to do some Activities if you are sitting on your own reading, but not all of them. Many of the Activities give you something to go out and try in practice. You are more likely to do them if, for example:

- You are going to talk to other people about them – your tutor/counsellor or colleagues
- You are interested enough to have a conversation with yourself about them – what the Russian psychologist Vygotsky called 'internalised dialogue'
- You decide to save them up for later, when you have more time.

If you want to do an Activity, give yourself enough time and plan:

- When you are going to do it
- What else you will need, apart from time; for example, you might have to do some research or talk to a few people
- How you will keep a record of what you have done – this is so you can look at it later, or include it in your profile.

Reflection sometimes requires you to stand back from what you have been doing and make a deliberate effort to think about it. Talking or writing can help.

Think, talk or write about:

- What you just did, for example, tackled an Activity on your own, read a Section of the book, tried to talk to somebody
- Why you did it like that
- Where it seems to fit in with what you have done before
- What was good and bad about it
- How you felt about it
- What it made you think.

What are the consequences?

- Describe the situation
- Ask yourself why it happened the way it did
- Think about how it was different from what you expected
- Work out what to do next.

You may want to keep track of what you have read in the book. Devise a system of marking the book to help you keep track.There is a box next to each heading on the contents page which you could tick when you have read the topic. Or you could highlight the boxes to show which topics you want to investigate in more depth.

Apollinaire said
'Come to the edge'
'But it is too high'
'Come to the edge'
'We might fall'
'Come to the edge'
And they came
And he pushed them
And they flew

You might decide to keep an Activity log as a record of your intentions and what you achieved by doing the Activities.

Integrating learning into practice

As you study this unit, or the degree programme as a whole, you will be learning general things as well as specific knowledge related to the unit topics. Your learning should integrate into practice. Many descriptions of the professional role emphasise the importance of continual learning. One study looking at the links between degree-level education and practice (Winter, 1994) identified that the professional role includes these four things:

- A requirement that understanding should continually develop through reflection upon practice
- Interpretative responsibility towards an always incomplete body of knowledge
- A basis in a complex set of ethical principles
- An understanding of the importance of affective dimensions (conscious and unconscious)

Another study looking at evidence of capability in a professional context (Eraut, 1994) found that the professional role includes:

- Understanding clients
- Analysing problems and situations
- Discussing the relative merits of alternative approaches
- Evaluating the professional practice you observe
- Conceptualising and evaluating your own work in order to learn from experience
- Creating knowledge.

The study also emphasised the value of underlying knowledge of techniques (including those still at pilot stage) and critical understanding of:

- The concepts, theories and principles which underpin current practice
- The significance of innovations
- The role played by your profession in society.

What does being a professional mean to you?

You might like to compare your thoughts with those expressed in the literature issued by your relevant statutory, professional or self-regulating body.

'When a practitioner becomes a researcher into his own practice, he engages in a continuing process of self-education.' Schön, D. (1991) *The Reflective Practitioner: How professionals think in action.* Aldershot, Hants: Avebury Press.

'"I didn't realise I knew so much. I didn't realise I do so much". This is the sort of statement often made by people who have spent some time evaluating their jobs.' Hull, C. (1992) Making experience count: facilitating the APEL process. In: Griffin, C. and Mulligan, J. (eds). *Empowerment Through Experiential Learning.* London: Kogan Page.

Do you have an appropriate sense of what you do and what you know?

Use a journal or reflective diary as a way of evaluating what you do and what you need to know in order to do it.

Assessment guidelines

This unit can be used to gain credits towards a BSc degree programme. To gain credit you will need to do some work that can be assessed. It is a good idea to start thinking about assessment right now. *You* can take charge of assessment – within the limits of the BSc programme and what you agree with your tutor/counsellor after negotiation.

If you wish to undertake the degree you will need to show that you can:

- Critically reflect on and challenge existing practice
- Draw on perspectives from within and beyond your own professional boundaries and use these to inform your own practice, where appropriate
- Develop and extend your own professional knowledge and skills through a process of analysis, synthesis and evaluation of the contemporary theoretical concepts that underpin current practice
- Plan, conduct and evaluate an enquiry-based project related to your field of practice
- Critically reflect on and evaluate your own personal, professional development and learning.

These are the overall learning outcomes for the degree as a whole. You should demonstrate that you have achieved them all throughout your work on the degree, including the unit assessments and the enquiry-based project.

The specific learning outcomes for this unit require you to:

- Critically evaluate the spectrum of approaches to enquiry and their application to the field of healthcare practice
- Justify the selection of approaches and methods used for the independent enquiry in an aspect of professional practice
- Plan, implement, critically evaluate and reflect on the process of completing a sustained independent enquiry into an aspect of professional practice
- Develop recommendations based upon a critical analysis of the findings of the enquiry.

To gain credits towards the degree, you will need to produce a written assessment which shows that you have achieved all the learning outcomes. In the assessment you will write a report of the independent enquiry which you have undertaken into an aspect of professional practice. It is up to you to decide on a topic for

There is a game about assessment with five stages. Playing the game shows what it is like when you can negotiate the assessment process. It is played in a group of 12 or more.

Stage 1 – One person is asked to stand up and clap, then leave the room.

Stage 2 – Four or five people are given a clapping score sheet and asked to act as an assessment panel. They have to decide individual criteria for assessing how well people clap. Next, another person is asked to stand up and clap, and then leaves the room. Each member of the panel awards the clapper a score out of five.

Stage 3 – Members of the panel get together to agree their criteria for assessing how well people clap. The next person is asked to stand up and clap and leaves the room while the panel agrees what score to award. The clapper is told the score but is not told what it means.

Stage 4 – The next person is told the criteria before being asked to clap. That person is also told the final score, together with an explanation.

Stage 5 – The last clapper is asked to sit down and have a chat about clapping. The panel acknowledges that the clapper has some knowledge of the subject and they ask what criteria the clapper would like to be assessed against. The criteria are agreed and the person is asked to clap when ready. The clapper is asked for an opinion of the performance. After a brief discussion, the panel then describes how they would assess the performance and a final score is negotiated by the panel and the clapper.

How do you think each of the clappers in the game described above might feel?

Which one would you rather be?

What do you think the game shows about different ways of assessing performance?

your enquiry. Negotiate with your tutor/counsellor the exact wording of your project title.

The enquiry-based project is a major piece of research including a written assessment. This unit gives you guidance on how to carry out the project. Your work on other units may give you ideas for topics to cover in the enquiry-based project. Talk to your tutor/counsellor about any practical details to do with assessment and refer for guidance to the university's regulations which accompany these materials.

Developing an idea for a project

At first, you may not have a clear idea of a topic for enquiry. However, you should start developing your ideas as early as you can. The book offers plenty of guidance. When you feel that you have the germ of an idea, start talking about it with other people – healthcare professionals, friends, your tutor/counsellor. If you don't feel ready to talk to other people, have a conversation – or several conversations – with yourself. Or write things down in your learning journal or reflective diary.

Don't worry if your ideas change a lot. But, sooner or later, you should put them down on paper and start to define the subject and scope of your assessment. Then negotiate the exact wording of the assessment with your tutor/counsellor.

The assessment habit

Get into the habit of assessing your work on this unit. Assessing yourself isn't only about deciding a topic for enquiry and completing the written assessment. People assess themselves all the time, often without realising it. They assess their behaviour, their moods, the way other people see them, the way they do things . . . One of the purposes of assessment is to help you learn, to clarify your reasons for learning certain things and to gauge how far you are getting. It can give you:

- Motivation – a reason for learning
- Practice – the opportunity to try things out
- Feedback – other people's comments on how you are doing
- Opportunity for reflection – time to think about what you have learned and how you have learned it, so as to build new knowledge into your existing practice.

Educational assessment is one of many forms of assessment which go on all the time. When you bake a cake you assess its success – how it looks, how it tastes, whether people like it. When you have a conversation you assess how the other person is responding to what you say. Derek Rowntree identifies the following, more formal kinds of assessment in addition to everyday conversational dialogue:

- Medical diagnosis
- The writing of biography
- Forensic cross-questioning
- Job interviews and promotion appraisals
- Criticism of the arts
- Refereeing of books and papers submitted for publication by scholarly journals.

'Such forms of assessment will sometimes offer revealing parallels and contrasts with those common in education.' Rowntree, D. (1977) *Assessing Students: How shall we know them?* London: Kogan Page.

You can negotiate a topic for your enquiry-based project with your tutor/counsellor. It is important that the topic allows you to demonstrate your understanding of the theory underpinning your work and to meet the learning outcomes.

Examples of appropriate projects include:

- A piece of action research
- A substantial literature review and critical analysis
- A field study based on gathering empirical data
- A feasibility study
- An in-depth review using critical incident techniques.

The personal profile

Assessment in the wider sense helps to keep track of your personal and professional development during your studies. One way of capturing parts of this process is to keep a personal profile. The profile can provide you with a rich source of reflective material to be drawn on when planning and producing the written assessment. Use the profile to record your thoughts about how learning and assessment fit together.

The profile can draw on all your experiences and encompass many different kinds of writing. If you are keeping a learning journal, reflective diary or activity log, they can form part of the profile. This kind of informal writing will help you to articulate what Donald Schön calls 'knowing in action' (Schön, 1987). It also gives you the chance to use your imagination to look at different possibilities without having to risk trying things out in reality.

Writing, reflection and learning feed into one another. As you examine your work, writing your thoughts down will help you to make connections between learning, feeling and doing. This kind of informal writing helps you discover what you think about complex topics and will help you write better formal assessments.

What is profiling?

Profiling helps you (and others) make sense of what you are learning and relate it to your professional and personal life. It is a structured approach for reflecting on:

- Yourself
- Your abilities
- Different aspects of your life and work – including your career and professional development to date
- Plans for the future.

It will help you:

- Understand the complexity of your work
- Analyse your experience and view it more critically
- Appreciate your own professional development
- Value the extent of your learning.

Profiling means keeping a record of these things, organised in a way that is clear to you. Most profiles include a fair bit of writing, because this is a good way of keeping a record and because writing things down often helps you clarify them in your mind. Writing can also help you make connections between different aspects of your life and learning.

There are many different names for the things which make up a profile, for example:

- A learning journal
- A reflective diary
- An activity log
- A reading log
- An action planner...

It doesn't matter what you call things as long as you write regularly and keep track of your thoughts and ideas.

What do you understand by the term 'critically reflect'? Draw on perspectives from outside your own professional boundaries when you are thinking about this question.

What do you understand by words such as 'synthesis' and 'evaluation'?

Where can you go to share ideas about questions such as these?

Reflection involves 'creating stops in which one stands aside from one's own process and has a look to see what is happening.' Brazier, D. (1995) *Zen Therapy*. London: Constable.

Find time every so often to let your thoughts catch up with you. Give them a bit of space inside your head and let them speak to you. One of the good things about learning is that, given the chance, you will discover new thoughts that have formed themselves without your even knowing it.

'I shall be telling this with a sigh,

Somewhere ages and ages hence:

Two roads diverged in a wood, and I –

I took the one less travelled by,

And that has made all the difference.'

Frost, R. (1951) 'The Road Not Taken'. *The Complete Poems of Robert Frost*, London: Jonathan Cape.

You will find suggestions on how to write things down, and where, as you work through this book; for example, in learning journals, reflective diaries, activity logs.

Other ways of keeping a record and thinking things through include drawing, taking photographs and recording on cassette significant conversations with other people. These can all form part of a profile and can be a good alternative to different forms of writing.

Whose profile is it?
Your personal profile is mainly for you. It will be a unique record of you as a learner. This means that you have control over where to start and what to include. There are no right or wrong ways. Some people prefer to start by keeping a reflective diary. Others start with a record of their professional education and training. Before you work on your profile you might find it useful to discuss it with a colleague, friend or tutor/counsellor. Identifying the different ways of using your profile will help you decide where and how you would like to start.

You may want to show some of it to other people as well. For example, if you have been thinking through a particular aspect of your work or your assessment, you may want to photocopy your notes, diagrams and ideas and discuss them with your tutor/counsellor or colleagues.

Macmillan Open Learning publishes a profile pack and workbook giving guidance on how to keep and use a profile. The handbook called *A Student's Guide to Open Learning* also contains a section on profiling. Both are available from Macmillan Open Learning at the address listed on page 2.

Profiling will help you as an individual to:
- Understand and appreciate the significance of what and how you learn
- Enhance your self-awareness and build confidence in the value of your experiences.

Profiling will help you as a professional to:
- Keep an effective and up-to-date record of your past and current learning
- Provide you with a powerful means of communication with your employers, present and future.

Think about keeping track of your reading in a learning journal. Whenever you read a book, a newspaper or journal article, write down your response to what you have read, any ideas which caught your imagination, questions that arose, further reading to be done. Your reading does not need to be confined to your subject area. Follow your interests and read widely. Parts of your journal might give you ideas for your written assessment.

Here are some guidelines for keeping track of reading:

- Read and write with some purpose in mind. Say why you selected a book or an article and what, overall, you learned from it, before taking issue with particular content
- Focus on things which strike you or are intriguing to you in some way.

Nightingale, P. (1986) *Improving Student Writing.* Kensington, New South Wales: Higher Education Research and Development Society of Australasia.

There could be two types of material in your profile:

- Confidential – that which is for your eyes only
- Professional – information about your learning and professional development that you are happy to share with others.

If you have started a profile for other purposes, you can continue using it for this unit.

Learning contracts

A learning contract is the sort of contract you can continually revise. It is not a binding legal document. The idea of a contract is to set out an agreement between two or more people – in this case, you and your tutor/counsellor. One of the things about a contract is that it helps you clarify your ideas, select realistic objectives and keep track of changes. Contracts don't have to be written down, although they usually are because writing down what you are intending to do is likely to help you develop planning and writing skills.

The work you do in your personal profile should lead you towards making a learning contract. As you think about what you have done in the past and what you are doing now, your thoughts will move to the future. Most people have both short- and long-term goals. The profile is a good place to make notes of your plans and goals. Make these as specific as possible. You can refine them as you try new approaches and techniques. When you are happy, transfer them to the learning contract. If you use action plans as well, you have a very good system for monitoring your progress. If you find yourself straying too far from your goals, make some adjustments, both to your course and to your contract.

There is no one right way to construct a learning contract. People learn and speak and write in different ways. You might have to try out several approaches before finding the one that suits you best. On the page opposite you will see two different approaches.

'It is important to remember that no one has the right to read your portfolio without your permission. The UKCC reminds registrants that "your portfolio contains confidential information about you and should, therefore, not be accessible to others without your permission".

'When deciding whether to give your permission, you need to understand the person's reasons for wanting to read your portfolio. Knowing the reason behind their request will enable you to select parts of your portfolio that are relevant to their interest.'

Hull, C. and Redfern, E. (1996) *Profiles and Portfolios. A guide for nurses and midwives.* Basingstoke: Macmillan.

A lifeline (or road of life) is a picture of your professional and/or personal life. It shows both highs and lows as well as important events. It can contain a little or a lot of information.

Draw a road of life showing how you came to be doing this unit or the degree programme.

- How are events related?
- Where are the turning points?

As you go through the programme, think about how it is affecting your professional and personal life.

- What causes the highs?
- At what points do the lows occur?

Keep drawing the line as you go through the programme, and afterwards.

LEARNING CONTRACT

Re: Section 2

What do I need to do?

1 Use the next three weeks to work through the unit.
2 Plan time in my diary to visit the library to follow up references.
3 Attend group tutorial.
4 Make one appointment with tutor/counsellor to discuss ideas I have about my assessment.

What am I trying to learn from this section?

(to be discussed with t/c after group tutorial)

1 The various models for structured reflection, especially Johns:
   - Making notes from the materials
   - Trying things out
   - Asking Jenny (fellow student) if she'll let me try and explain it to her
2 I'd really like to find out whether reflection works in practice — I'll aim to experiment with critical incident analysis.

LEARNING CONTRACT

This is the first time I've ever learnt this way and I keep getting lost and feeling I'm not achieving anything. A colleague suggested I make a definite plan – what I'm going to learn and then agree it with my tutor/counsellor. I decided to try it for Sections 1 and 2.

1 Go through, page by page, and mark up any references I need to follow up.
   Action: Book time to go to the library.
2 Not sure about the difference between different models of reflection. Is there a real difference or is it just words?
   Action: Need to explore this with colleagues.
3 I've really been thinking about why I'm involved in health care.
   Action: Write a mission statement for myself as an hcp.
4 Concept analysis seems a bit complex.
   Action: Phone t/c to talk about some ideas and check whether I've got it right.
5 Need to learn about how really to read and evaluate articles I find. It's difficult to know whether they are right or wrong about what they're saying.
   Action: Need to think about how I can do that.

Remember these general principles for evidence of your learning:

- Relevance – your learning must be relevant to the subject you are aiming to study or the award you are seeking
- Breadth – the learning you are demonstrating should relate to a wide body of knowledge and skills, particularly in the context of your own professional practice
- Currency – the learning you are showing must be up to date and relevant to your current working practices
- Authenticity – the evidence you provide must be your own work.

When assessing your life and learning, the following elements are involved:

- Your learning and your experience
- Reflecting upon your past learning
- Identifying significant learning
- Providing evidence of learning
- Direct evidence – things you produce yourself
- Indirect evidence – things other people say on your behalf.

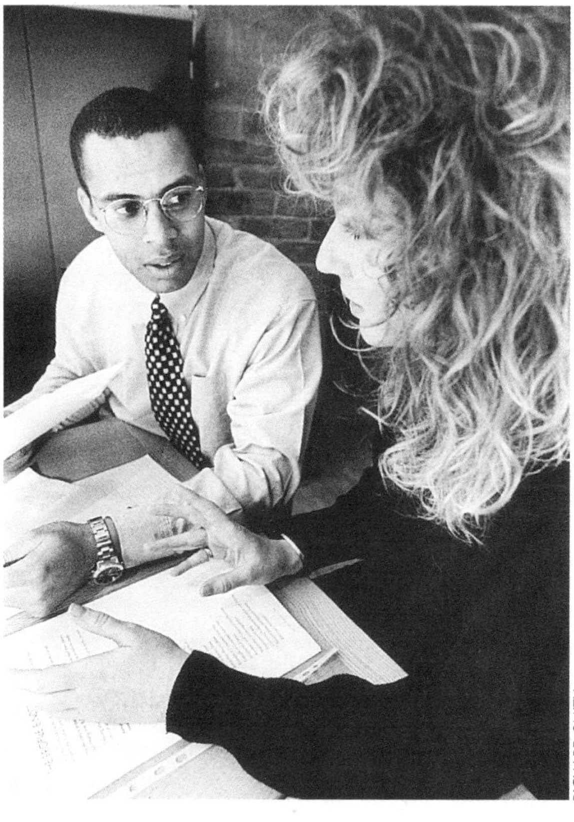

RICHARD SMITH

Enquiring into practice

You learn something new every day. As you do your job, you are constantly refining and improving your practice – discovering how to complete a particular procedure more smoothly, gaining new insight into a familiar situation, or developing your skills in other ways. Most of this learning happens in small, unconnected pieces, building up over time into the 'experience' that sets you apart from new recruits to your profession.

This unit offers you some tools which you can use to organise and intensify your learning. You can use this unit while undertaking a formal enquiry-based project on which you will be assessed. The ideas and techniques you meet here should also prove stimulating and useful in your everyday work. As an added benefit, you may find that the process of discovering how an enquiry-based project is planned and carried out will make the work of other researchers and enquirers more interesting and accessible to you.

The concepts of enquiry and research may seem far removed from the day-to-day work with which you are familiar. But this need not be the case. In fact, the closer the topic you choose to investigate is to your everyday work, the better.

The more personally concerned you are with your topic, the more insight and knowledge you will bring to it. Your enquiry could stem from positive or negative feelings about your present practice. You may want to investigate a promising new approach – or find a solution to a problem. Or you might simply want to explore an area of your work which you believe is inadequately understood.

Several methods of enquiry are presented in this unit. The first techniques described are intended to help you develop your skills as a reflective practitioner. By learning to detach yourself from a situation and reflect on what is really going on, you may gain some refreshing new perspectives.

The unit goes on to describe how to conduct a literature search. This will help you find out what is already known about the topic you are interested in. You will discover how understanding has developed over recent years and what the current state of knowledge is. A well-organised and comprehensive literature search and review can be of enormous value in suggesting or clarifying a topic for enquiry. Or you may decide to collect your own primary data. This could involve making observations, or

Why do healthcare practitioners need to undertake research and enquiry?

'There are a number of reasons why any clinician, not only an occupational therapist, should *want* to do research, and should actually be *doing* research. The first is that it's stimulating; the second that it's part of good clinical practice; and the third that it's a valuable form of quality assurance of a clinical service.'

Brooks, N. (1988) Why research? *British Journal of Occupational Therapy* 51: 11: 397–398.

The following is an outline of the contents of each Section of this book

Section 1– What are you going to investigate?

This Section asks you to reflect on your practice and select a topic to investigate in your enquiry. Several tools for reflection are introduced, including critical incident analysis and three models of structured reflection.

Section 2 – Methods of enquiry

This Section discusses research methods and how they differ from the informal methods of enquiry in everyday life. It describes different approaches to research and the perspectives which underlie them.

perhaps conducting a survey or series of in-depth interviews.

Whatever form your enquiry takes, it is important that you gather and present your information in such a way that it is of use to other professionals. This is where the methods of enquiry come in. You will find out about the rules and conventions which give authority to your work and allow other people to evaluate your findings. These conventions differ, depending on the type of enquiry you are doing. For example, in a survey, the way you choose your sample and ask your questions will influence the answers you get. If you are conducting an in-depth interview, quite different conventions and procedures are appropriate. You will also learn how to write up your report, so that other people will take it seriously.

We hope that you will find this unit useful in developing your own practice. In addition, by presenting your findings in a form that can be used by your colleagues, you will be contributing to the development of your profession.

References

Eraut, M. (1994) Implications for standards development. In: *Competence and Assessment Compendium No. 3.* London: Department of Employment.

Schön, D. (1987) *Educating the Reflective Practitioner.* San Francisco: Jossey-Bass.

Winter, R. (1994) The ASSET Programme – Competence-based education at professional/honours degree level. In: *Competence and Assessment Compendium No. 3.* London: Department of Employment.

Key texts for this unit

Bell, J. (1993) *Doing Your Research Project.* (2nd edition). Milton Keynes: Open University Press.

Boud, D., Keogh, R. and Walker, D. (1985) *Reflection: Turning experience into learning.* London: Kogan Page.

Carr, W. and Kemmis, S. (1986) *Becoming Critical.* London: Falmer Press.

Hicks, C.M. (1988) *Practical Research Methods for Physiotherapists.* Edinburgh: Churchill Livingstone.

Palmer, A., Burns, S. and Bulman, C. (1994) *Reflective Practice in Nursing – The growth of the professional practitioner.* Oxford: Blackwell Scientific.

Polit, D. and Hungler, B. (1993) *Essentials of Nursing Research* (3rd ed.). Philadelphia: J.B. Lippincott Company.

Reason, P. (1988) *Human Inquiry in Action.* London: Sage Publications.

Schön, D.A. (1991) *The Reflective Turn – Case studies in and on educational practice.* New York: Teachers' College Press.

Tripp, D. (1993) *Critical Incidents in Teaching.* London: Routledge.

Winter, R. (ed) (1989) *Learning from Experience – Principles and practice in action research.* London: Falmer Press.

Section 3 – Exploring the literature

This Section explains how to conduct a literature search and describes some techniques you could use when reading books and journals and when taking notes. It also contains guidelines for reading research reports and an introduction to understanding statistical information.

Section 4 – Planning and carrying out your enquiry

This Section describes the stages of the research process, including the decisions to be taken at each of the stages. It provides more details about the procedures used in various forms of research.

Section 5 – Writing up your project

This Section provides information on the structure, layout and language of research reports. It also contains suggestions which may help you with the writing process and ideas about other ways of presenting your findings to different audiences.

Introduction

There may not be many opportunities in your professional life to spend time investigating an issue you have chosen for yourself. Your independent enquiry-based project is a rare and valuable chance to explore or extend an aspect of practice. This Section aims to help you make the most of the opportunity by helping you choose a topic that is important to you.

You might, for example, decide to base your project on:

- Something you find challenging - such as methods of assessing levels of pain in young children
- Something you would like to know more about - such as the health beliefs of a particular cultural group
- Something you think could be done more effectively - such as admission procedures.

The topic you choose could be relevant to your day-to-day work, but it need not be. You don't have to go for an obviously relevant topic. For example, if you are working with people with diabetes you may not get much chance in your work to investigate those with HIV/AIDS. But if that is what interests you, think how it might be possible to carry out an enquiry in this area.

Whatever topic you choose, it should be central to your own values and priorities as a healthcare professional - and as a person.

This Section offers you some reflective and analytical tools to help you:

- Identify where your concerns and interests lie
- Choose an appropriate topic for your project.

From time to time, you may like to use techniques such as critical incident analysis or guided reflection to help you choose and define your topic for enquiry. These are discussed later in this Section. Many of the techniques introduced here will be useful throughout your work on the project, not just at the start.

'. . . an important minority of nurses are still debating the value of research and its use in the delivery of care. Many more nurses realise that research is the basis for clinical care and that areas of clinical concern should point the way for future research, but are not quite sure how this can be achieved. Those nurses who are comfortable combining research findings with clinical practice would appear to be in a minority.'

Chapman, H. (1996) Why do nurses not make use of a solid research base? *Nursing Times* 92:(3): 38-39.

Does the comment from Chapman in the box on the left about the attitude of nurses towards research hold true for your profession?

Why do you think it might be difficult to integrate research-based theory and practice?

What does health care mean to you?

The topic you choose to investigate in your project should be central to your own priorities and values. There are several benefits in selecting a topic in which you have a genuine interest:

- Your motivation to study will be increased
- Your existing knowledge and experience will make it easier for you to understand the literature
- You may have personal insights and understanding which can add depth to your research
- Your research project may open doors to new areas of work for you.

RICHARD SMITH

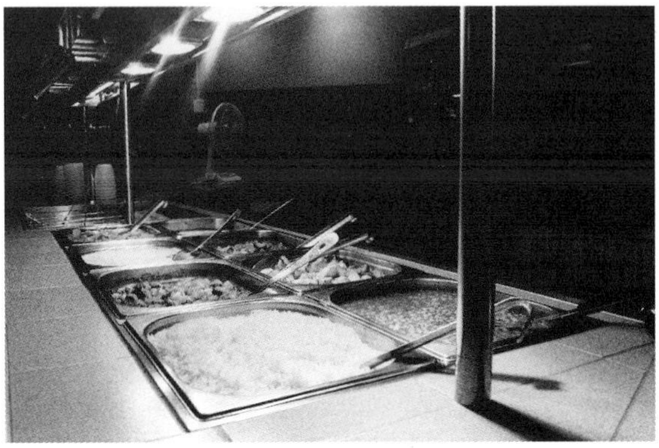

What topics of enquiry are there in this?

DEPARTMENT OF HEALTH

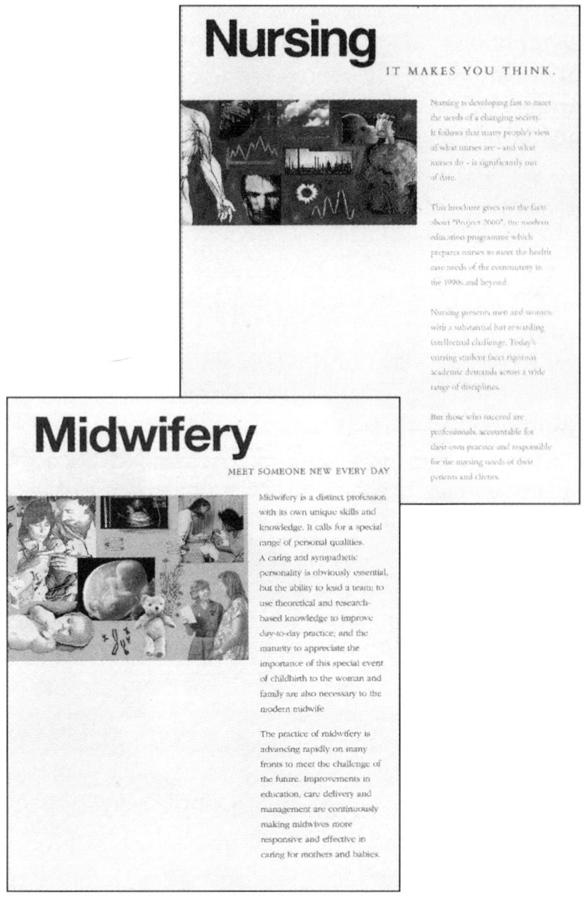

Nursing

IT MAKES YOU THINK.

Nursing is developing fast to meet the needs of a changing society. It follows that many people's view of what nurses are – and what nurses do – is significantly out of date.

This brochure gives you the facts about "Project 2000", the modern education programme which prepares nurses to meet the health care needs of the community in the 1990s and beyond.

Nursing presents men and women with a substantial but rewarding intellectual challenge. Today's nursing student faces rigorous academic demands across a wide range of disciplines.

But those who succeed are professionals, accountable for their own practice and responsible for the nursing needs of their patients and clients.

Midwifery

MEET SOMEONE NEW EVERY DAY

Midwifery is a distinct profession with its own unique skills and knowledge. It calls for a special range of personal qualities. A caring and sympathetic personality is obviously essential, but the ability to lead a team; to use theoretical and research-based knowledge to improve day-to-day practice; and the maturity to appreciate the importance of this special event of childbirth to the woman and family are also necessary to the modern midwife

The practice of midwifery is advancing rapidly on many fronts to meet the challenge of the future. Improvements in education, care delivery and management are continuously making midwives more responsive and effective in caring for mothers and babies.

When you have a dialogue, it doesn't have to be with someone you actually know. You could think of anyone you would like to meet - perhaps someone you admire or a character from a film or a book.

What would it be like to talk to this person? Imagine the atmosphere in the room. Think about how the conversation with the person might go if you told them what matters to you about your work. Have an imaginary discussion with the person in your head.

Explain to an imaginary child why you are doing your job. Tape-record or write down what you say. Reflect on your explanation.

- How convincing is it?
- Is it related to daily reality?
- What questions might an awkward child ask about what you say – and how would you answer?

The positive images above of nursing and midwifery have been used in recruitment literature published by the Department of Health.

- If you were advising a 16-year-old who was considering training for the job you are doing now, what else would you want them to know?
- What kinds of pictures would you use to show what your work is like?
- In what way (if any) would they be different from the pictures used in the recruitment leaflets pictured above?

You might want to start a collection of pictures relating to your own area of practice, illustrating positive and negative aspects of your work.

If you are undertaking the degree programme, think about which of the other units you are studying are the most stimulating.

- Can you explain why they interest you most?
- Would you like to find out more about the issues and questions they raise?

Values

Most healthcare professionals find that the everyday demands of their work take up a lot of attention and energy. It can be difficult to stop and consider underlying values and perhaps to remember the hopes and expectations with which they started out in the profession. Ideas of this kind may even seem naïve and idealistic once they are aware of the complexities of working life. Even so, it is important that people do not lose sight of what they hold to be valuable and significant about the work they do.

Your project offers you an opportunity to explore these values and to investigate how you can embody them more effectively in your day-to-day practice.

Here are two examples:

A practice nurse felt that her major contribution was in the area of health promotion. She felt that the most significant lifestyle change people could make was to give up smoking, and had started running anti-smoking classes. But take-up was not encouraging, so she decided to base her research project on methods of improving attendance at classes of this kind.

A children's nurse felt strongly that many young people below the age of consent should be allowed more say in important decisions about their treatment. She decided to investigate law and practice in this area.

Here is a mind map which a healthcare professional started to draw in order to explore what health care meant for her:

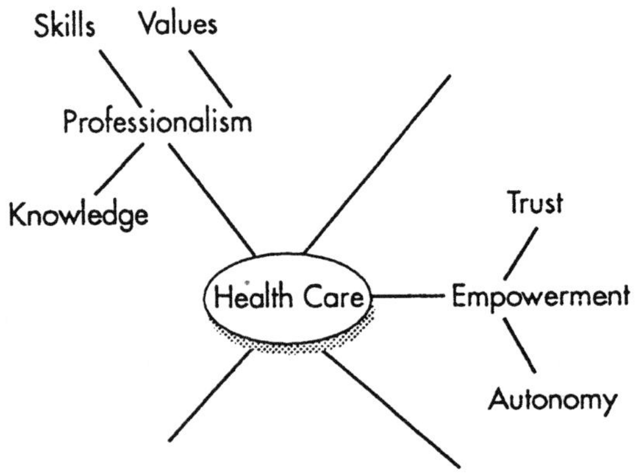

Answer the questions below quickly, without thinking too much about them. Write down short, one-or two-line answers.

- What do you find most satisfying about your job?
- What do you find most irritating about it?
- What do you find most challenging about it?
- Where do you think you, personally, could make your most significant contribution?
- What aspect of your job would you change, if you were able to?

Come back to the questions and your answers in a few days' time. Would you answer them in the same way?

Identify an aspect of your practice you would like to change.

- What obstacle lies between you and your goal - is it knowledge, resources, or something else?
- Is there any way in which your project could provide a stepping stone towards your goal?

It is as well to choose an area of research that is related to your everyday practice. It is also important that your research topic is personally significant. The Activities on these two pages offer you a chance to step back and think about what really matters to you in your job.

The day-to-day reality

Another way of identifying an area to explore in your project is to focus consciously on the day-to-day reality of work. Instead of taking the 'macro' view, as you were encouraged to do in the Activities on the previous two pages, take a 'micro' view and examine the minutiae of what you do in your job.

You are probably familiar with the technique in which a hidden camera is used, with the knowledge and consent of participants, to observe the interactions of clients such as parents and children. The videotape is then reviewed, analysed and discussed — and can provoke remarkable insights. For example, the mother of a young child with cerebral palsy complained that she was having tremendous difficulty in feeding her daughter. When she watched herself on video, she was able to see that she was rushing the child and not making adequate allowance for her daughter's underdeveloped swallowing reflex.

The Activities on this page suggest similar techniques that you can use to consider your own work.

Because of the ethical and practical problems involved, you probably should not video yourself at work. But it is possible to make a detailed record of events in other ways.

If you can make an objective record of exactly what you do, you may discover, for example:

- Habits you were not aware of
- Discrepancies from what you think you do
- How your actions are perceived by others
- How you might do certain things more effectively.

For example, a physiotherapist working in an orthopaedic ward recorded the number of times she went to speak to each of the patients in her care during a shift. She discovered that she spent more of her time with younger patients and very little with older patients who had some sensory loss, and with whom she found it difficult to communicate.

Write down everything that happened in an hour during your previous day at work. Imagine yourself as a camera, recording everything you see and hear.

Next time you go to work, keep the 'camera' running for an hour. Does it make you more aware of what is going on around you?

'The easiest way for me to see myself is in images. Images of flowers, in Winnie the Pooh, sea gulls. I don't know if I could ever do it using words. A lot of times you see something in your own mind. Other times you see it and there's no word connection. It's . . . bonk . . . and it's there and it's really a true form of understanding. It's hard to use words.'

Women's Ways of Knowing. The development of self, voice and mind. Belenky, M.F., Clinchy, B.M., Goldberger, N.R., Tarule, J.M. (1986). London: Basic Books, distributed by HarperCollins.

Cricket has been likened to chess - batsmen in cricket analyse the way they hit the ball in the same way as chess players analyse their moves. Cricket statisticians use diagrams like the one below to record where the batsman hits the ball in an innings. Other cricketers can then use the information to work out where a particular player's strengths and weaknesses lie and to plan their strategy.

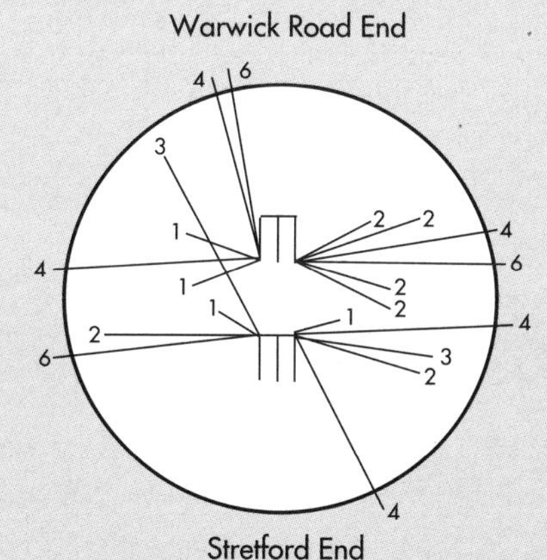

How could this suggest ways of analysing aspects of what you do? What could you draw?

Other people's perspectives
It can be very instructive to look at your own actions from a different perspective. One way to do this is to think about how the situation looks to 'a fly on the wall'. It may tell you a great deal about how people interact with each other. Or you could try to take the viewpoint of another individual involved in a situation. For example, put yourself in the place of someone using the health service or another member of staff, as did this nurse in an accident and emergency ward:

'I thought it was perfectly reasonable to ask the receptionist to telephone a patient's partner and was annoyed when it took her over half an hour to make the call. When I watched her working, however, I realised that she was constantly dealing with incoming calls, questions from patients and requests for information from other members of the nursing and medical staff. By changing my perspective, I gained a valuable insight into my own working relationship with this colleague.'

Look for a meaning
Looking at the details of what happens in your workplace will almost certainly reveal much wider issues which could become the topic of your project.

You may like to focus on an area which you are aware is significant. Perhaps you have already identified a problem, or an incident that gave you particular satisfaction. You might also be conscious that you always react in a similar way when a certain situation arises at work.
It can sometimes be interesting to look in detail at an incident or procedure which, at first sight, doesn't seem very significant. Things which are done automatically do not, by definition, receive much analysis. When you do study them in detail, you may be surprised at what you find.

Pages 22 and 23 show how you can use the technique of critical incident analysis to draw out general issues from particular situations.

When a stage play is in rehearsal, the actors' moves may be 'mapped out' in diagrams to show where they should go on the stage.

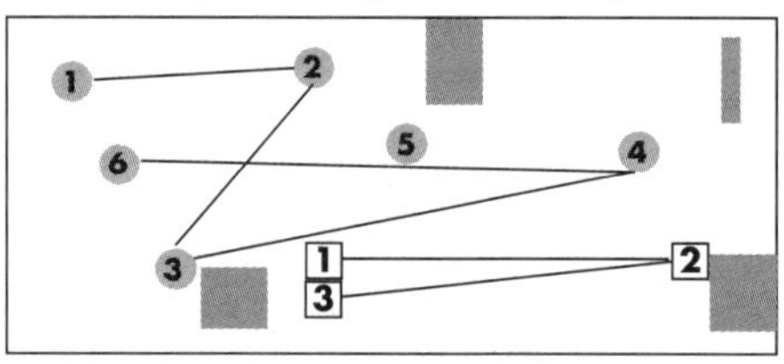

If you used a similar technique to record how people move around the area in which you work, what might it reveal?

'What can be expressed in words can be expressed in life.'
Thoreau, H. D. from a letter to H. G. O. Blake, March 27, 1848.
Quoted in: Thomas, B. (1994) *If Monks had Macs.* New York: Voyager.

The unit entitled *Professional Relationships: Influences on health care* looks at the wider issues involved in working with other people.

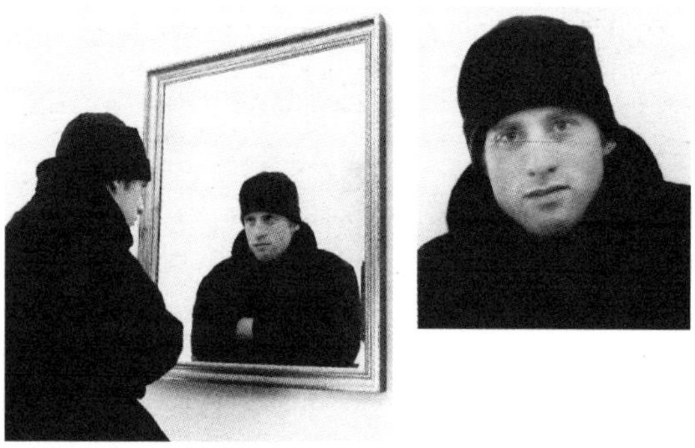

RICHARD SMITH

Different camera shots give different types of information. Next time you watch a TV drama, notice how the camera moves and uses different techniques to show what is going on in a particular situation.

- When you look at things, do you naturally take a 'wide shot' of everything that is going on, or do you 'zoom in' and take 'close-ups' of the action immediately in front of you?
- How can thinking like this about your own ways of looking help you decide on a topic for enquiry?

Using the reflective process in enquiry

Reflection is central to all techniques for recording and thinking about experience. It is a method of enquiry in itself and you will find yourself using it as you think of ideas for your project and when you are carrying it out.

On the next six pages you will find more about the reflective process and how it can point out areas for examination and study.

To reflect upon something is to consider it carefully and calmly. Reflection involves separating yourself from your experience so that you can examine and evaluate it. Most of the time, people don't look at the world objectively. Their normal perception of events is subjective. They may be affected by, among other things:

- An underlying emotional state
- The emotional effect a particular event has on them
- Opinions and assumptions about what is going on
- Lack of understanding or knowledge.

All these influences form people's view of reality. It is only by becoming conscious of the subjective nature of perception that we can allow for it and see what is happening from other points of view.

For many people, emotions are the biggest block to objectivity. You can probably think of times when you have been upset by something and gone on to react inappropriately strongly to another, perhaps completely unrelated, event. It is quite normal to carry an 'emotional history' with you in your interactions with other people. For example, if you have had a good experience with a particular colleague or client in the past, you will bring positive expectations to your next encounter, and this will flavour your experience.

It can be more difficult to recognise some of the mental attitudes and assumptions you carry. People are often unconscious of some of these views and preconceptions. Reflection can allow them to take a long, cool look at the logic of their actions and can reveal some interesting 'blind spots'.

Children who visit the Eureka! museum in Halifax are invited to record their reactions to the exhibition by stamping their 'passport' with one of a series of faces:

Amazed	Puzzled
Curious	Disappointed
Excited	Worried
Happy	Bored

Draw cartoon faces to show:

- How you felt at the end of your last day at work
- How you felt the last time a client or a colleague thanked you for something you had done
- How you are feeling at this moment.

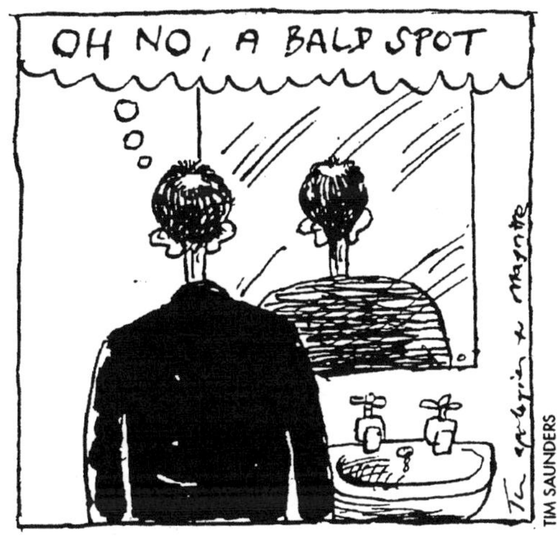

TIM SAUNDERS

'We do not see things as they are, but as we are.'
The Talmud

Reflection can make us aware of aspects of ourselves we do not normally see. The unit, *Professional Relationships: Influences on health care,* looks in more detail at how the unconscious shapes our responses to people and events.

Here is a summary of the reflective process (Boud et al., 1985):

1 Return to the experience:
- Consider how you were feeling
- Catalogue the events
- Do not give praise or criticism

2 Attend to feelings:
- Consider whether your present feelings about the experience are colouring your memory of it
- Consider what perceptions are blocking the analysis of events

3 Re-evaluate the experience:
- What really happened?
- How does it link with your own concept?
- What do you now know as a result?
- How do you feel about it?

You can go through the reflective process on your own, or you can ask someone else, such as a tutor/counsellor or a skilled and trusted friend, to guide you.

Other people can recognise and help you to acknowledge emotions and prejudices. In the absence of a helper, take some time to think about the points listed here and write down your responses to them. Go back to your notes later and see if you have any further thoughts. Critical incident analysis is a technique which can encourage this reflective process; for a more comprehensive definition see page 26. Together, these can lead you to a deeper appreciation of aspects of your work which you might want to investigate in more detail in your enquiry-based project.

Reflection on your own practice can be uncomfortable. You may discover things about yourself and the way you work that you don't find particularly admirable. If this happens, try to acknowledge what you are feeling. Use your reflective journal to record your feelings, and talk them over with someone you trust.

'As the professional moves towards new competences, he gives up some familiar sources of satisfaction and opens himself up to new ones. He gives up the rewards of unquestioned authority, the freedom to practise without challenge to his competence, the comfort of relative invulnerability, the gratifications of deference. The new satisfactions open to him are largely about his knowledge-in-practice, and about himself. When a practitioner becomes a researcher into his own practice, he engages in a continuing process of self-education.'

Schon, D. (1991)*The Reflective Practitioner. How professionals think in action.* Aldershot: Avebury Press.

'To leave the thread of all time
and let it make a dark line
in hopes that I can still find
the way back to the moment
I took the turn and turned to
begin a new beginning
still looking for the answer
I cannot find the finish
it's either this or that way
it's one way or the other
it should be one direction
it could be on reflection
the turn I have just taken
the turn I was just making
I might be just beginning
I might be near the end.'

'Anywhere is', a song from *The Memory of Trees* Album, by Enya. Warner Music UK Ltd.

The unit *Professional Relationships: Influences on health care,* deals with some of the difficulties of discovering new things about yourself.

Models of structured reflection — 1

These two pages and the next two introduce three models of structured reflection. Two of the models - those of Tripp, D. (1993) and Johns, C. (1994) - ask you to go beyond the reflections you make about yourself. They say that you should also consider the perceptions of other people and the effects of your actions on others. All three models are likely to highlight issues which need further investigation. You may find that these issues are suitable topics for your enquiry-based project.

The first model, shown opposite, was originally produced for use by school teachers. It provides a series of questions that can be used to examine a critical incident. You could use it as a day-to-day checklist for reflecting on everyday actions, or you could expand any of the questions to form the basis of a topic for more extended enquiry.

For example:

- The question: 'What does it feel like?' could become a study of the public's perceptions of a particular therapy
- The question: 'Why did (does) it occur?' could become an investigation of the public's reasons for not disclosing significant information to their professional carers.

An occupational therapist has this example:

'I used Tripp's model to look at an incident in which I was advising an elderly client on adaptations to her home which would increase her mobility. She was very uncommunicative and seemed uninterested in my efforts to make her life more comfortable - for example, she refused to look at brochures and plans. On reflection, I realised that this client had always been very proud of her house and the way it was decorated. For her, the installation of steps and hand rails represented a move towards 'institutionalisation' of her home. This got me thinking and I decided to use my project to investigate the aesthetic aspects of mobility aids.'

The box opposite 'How to create a critical incident' describes how an ordinary incident on a ward can become the starting point for a more general enquiry.

In the study quoted opposite, Jeff Dooley set out to find the answers to these questions:

- Can an individual acquire competence in reflection and enquiry skills through self-study?
- Is there a theory to guide us in acquiring that competence?
- If, like most people, we are not fully aware of the state of our own mental models, how can we progress through a programme of self-designed learning without being undermined by our inner defences?

There certainly aren't any easy answers to these questions. Just asking them may help you think about some of the reactions you will have when studying this unit and any problems you encounter.

A learning journal is a good place to note down your thoughts about general topics such as these.

'It's easy to espouse the principles of inquiry and reflection, but difficult to acquire a frame of mind which is open to this type of learning. . . . I found I had to combine study with regular practice . . . gradually we learned to inquire into the sources of each other's views, to catch ourselves when we tried to exert unilateral control over the conversation and to bring to the surface our long-cherished and secret, powerful, defensive routines.'

Dooley, J. (1994) Bootstrapping yourself into reflection and inquiry skills. In: Senge, P. (ed) *The Fifth Discipline Fieldbook.* London: Nicholas Brearley Publishing.

Questions used to examine a critical incident

Kind of judgement	*Information required*	*Questions asked*	*People involved*
Practical	Procedural	What should I do? How? When? Where?	For and/or with whom?
Diagnostic	Descriptive Causal Effectual Affectual Semantic Explanatory	What happened? What made it happen? What does it do? What does it feel like? What does it mean? Why did (does) it occur?	Who was involved? Who acted? For whom? For whom? To whom? With whom?
Reflective	Personal Evaluative	Do I like it? Is it a good thing?	Do others like it? For whom?

Tripp, D. (1993) *Critical Incidents in Teaching*. London: Routledge.

How to create a critical incident

Incident	Describe incident	Mrs M rang the bell and asked me to accompany her to the toilet
	Suggest explanation and meaning within the immediate context	It was what she was asked to do when she needed to go to the toilet It means that she is conforming to the rule that she should not leave her bed without telling a member of the nursing staff It is an example of the limits we put on the movements of some patients on the ward
Critical incident	Find a more general meaning and classification/significance of incident	Position: I think we put unnecessary limits on the movements of some patients

Based on Tripp, D. (1993) *Critical Incidents in Teaching*. London: Routledge.

Choose two incidents that have happened to you at work recently. One incident should be something that had an emotional impact on you. The other should be something trivial, about which you have no strong feelings. As you look through the model on this page and the two on the following pages, use them on your two incidents.

- How useful for your practice do you find each model?
- Do you find a particular model more appropriate for one incident than for the other? If so, why?
- What ideas do the models give you for your project?

Note your thoughts in your journal or diary.

Remember to be critical of everything you read in this book. Use your personal profile to record questions, comments or disagreements.

Models of structured reflection — 2

Like Tripp's model, which was described on page 23, John's model (shown below) asks questions about feelings. It also considers the background to the incident and factors which influence the way people act. An important feature of this model is that it asks you to think about:

- Alternative choices you could have made
- The implications of the experience for your own learning.

The last question in the model (question 5:4) refers to four patterns of knowing: empirical; aesthetic; ethical and personal. These categories relate to an influential theory by Carper (1978) which suggests that there are four distinct areas of knowledge needed by nurses:

- *Empirical:* this refers to the science of nursing - the kind of factual knowledge that can be verified by observation
- *Aesthetic:* this refers to the art of the practice of nursing - the ability to recognise what is significant in a patient's behaviour. It goes beyond a simple understanding of theory to its application in a particular situation
- *Ethical:* this refers to the moral component of nursing, which includes not only formal ethical codes but also all conscious actions
- *Personal:* this refers to the personal relationship which exists between nurse and patient.

Carper's four 'patterns of knowing' are considered in more detail later in Section 2, pp 52-53.

The third model, Mezirow's model, shown below opposite, divides reflection into two types (Mezirow, 1981):

- That which can lead to a change in perspective
- That which can be used to help us become more conscious and self-aware.

Mezirow encourages us to understand how personal history influences our behaviour in the present. The aim is that by using his model, we can achieve a degree of 'critical emancipation'.

According to Mezirow, there are four levels of reflection. First is a critical awareness of a particular situation. Next comes an awareness of our own feelings and patterns of thinking. The third level is the ability to discriminate between different ways of looking at the world that we may use - for example, many people behave very

The following cues are offered to help practitioners access, make sense of, and learn through experience.

1 Description
1.1 Write a description of the experiences
1.2 What are the key issues within this description that I need to pay attention to?

2 Reflection
2.1 What was I trying to achieve?
2.2 Why did I act as I did?
2.3 What were the consequences of my actions
- For the patient and family
- For myself
- For the people I work with

2.4 How did I feel about this experience when it was happening?
2.5 How did the patient feel about it?
2.6 How do I know how the patient felt about it?

3 Influencing factors
3.1 What internal factors influenced my decision-making and actions?
3.2 What external factors influenced my decision-making and actions?
3.3 What sources of knowledge did or should have influenced my decision-making and actions?

4 Could I have dealt better with the situation?
4.1 What other choices did I have?
4.2 What would be the consequences of these other choices?

5 Learning
5.1 How can I make sense of this experience in the light of past experience and future practice?
5.2 How do I NOW feel about this experience?
5.3 Have I taken effective action to support myself and others as a result of this experience?
5.4 How has this experience changed my ways of knowing in practice:
- empirical [What does it tell me about the science of nursing?]
- aesthetic [What does it tell me about the art of nursing?]
- ethical [What does it add to my understanding of moral issues?]
- personal [What does it add to my understanding of myself and my relationships with patients?]

Johns, C. (1994) Nuances of reflection. *Journal of Clinical Nursing* 3: 71-75.

differently when they are off duty. The final level is when we make conscious value judgements on the way we look at the world.

Mezirow's model also distinguishes between three forms of reflectivity, which refer to:
- The unconscious assumptions we make about the world
- Our own internal habits of thought and decision-making
- The theoretical basis which underpins our actions.

By understanding these we are in a better position to recognise the way people's actions are influenced by their beliefs. This understanding is a basis for learning.

Each of these levels of reflection and forms of reflectivity could suggest topics for your project.

A nurse came across the following note in her reflective diary:

'The charge nurse didn't seem to understand what the patient was asking him about until she spelt it out in words of one syllable. Typical male insensitivity! I knew PT was going to be difficult from the moment he came onto the ward. I don't think male nurses will be accepted by patients until they learn to empathise.'

What do you think this nurse could learn from applying Mezirow's three forms of reflectivity?

You might like to use Mezirow's model to formulate a series of questions which you can use to reflect upon your experience and suggest ideas for enquiry. Think about all three models.

What changes might you make to the models if you are interested in using them as part of your enquiry?

How might the changes affect the way you reflect on your own practice, and its effect on others?

Levels of reflection leading to perspective transformation

1. *Critical reflectivity*: becoming critically aware of a specific perception, meaning or behaviour of our own or of habits we have of seeing, thinking, feeling or acting.

2. *Affective reflectivity*: becoming aware of how we feel about the way we are perceiving, thinking or acting or about our habits of doing so.

3. *Discriminant reflectivity*: assessing the efficacy of our perceptions, thoughts, actions and habits of doing things, identifying immediate causes, recognising the context in which an incident took place (for example, playing, dreaming) and identifying our relationships in the situation.

4. *Judgemental reflectivity*: becoming aware of our value judgements about our perceptions, thoughts, habits and actions in terms of their being liked, disliked, beautiful or ugly, positive or negative.

Forms of reflectivity which lead to 'critical consciousness', and thus perspective transformation

Conceptual reflectivity: becoming conscious of our awareness and investigating the assumptions or constructs we are using to make decisions, ie what we are basing our decisions on and where we are coming from to arrive at these decisions

Psychic reflectivity: recognising in oneself the habit of making precipitant judgements about people on the basis of limited judgements about them, and recognising the interests and anticipations which influence the way we perceive, think or act.

Theoretical reflectivity: becoming aware that the theories that we hold, deeply espoused theories or taken-for-granted cultural or psychological assumptions, which explain personal experience less satisfactorily than other perspectives with more functional criteria for seeing, thinking or acting, are influencing our judgements.

Mezirow, J. (1981) Cited in Boud, D., Keogh, R and Walker, D. (1985) *Reflection: Turning experience into learning.* London: Kogan Page.

Critical incident analysis

Critical incidents were introduced on page 22 as a way of discovering aspects of practice which could be a starting point for an enquiry-based project. But how can you get to grips with incidents like these and explore the underlying issues they present?

The technique of critical incident analysis originated in the Second World War, when the US Army Air Force (USAF) need to select and train air crews quickly. Data available on why pilots failed the training programme were too vague to be useful, so instructors were asked to answer four questions about their trainees:

- When was the last time you saw a trainee pilot do something effective or ineffective?
- What led up to this situation?
- Exactly what did the trainee do?
- Why was it effective or ineffective?

The questions demanded factual answers - not intuitions or unfocused feelings about the general competence of particular individuals. Similar questions were asked of experienced pilots. In this way, the USAF built up a list of behaviours needed by pilots which could be used as the basis of a training programme.

Today, critical incident analysis is used by professionals in many fields, particularly as part of a reflective process. It can help identify the areas which professionals themselves recognise as critical. These incidents can then be grouped together and looked at in more depth.

'By an incident is meant any observable activity that is sufficiently complete in itself to permit inferences and predictions to be made about the person performing the act. To be critical, an incident must occur in a situation where the purpose of the act seems fairly clear to the observer and where its consequences are sufficiently definite to leave little doubt concerning its effects.' (Flanagan, 1954)

Here is an example of such an incident:

A midwife was performing a routine antenatal examination on a woman in the early stages of pregnancy. She told the woman that she would probably be able to listen to the fetal heartbeat, but, in fact, she was unable to locate it. The patient became alarmed and tearful. Although the midwife had no reason to suspect that there was anything amiss, she called in a doctor to assist in order to reassure the mother.

How would you apply the last three of the four original critical incident questions listed above to the actions of the midwife described above?

Choose a critical incident from your own practice. Apply the same three questions to it.

You can find out more about critical thinking by reading:

Brookfield, S. (1987) *Developing Critical Thinkers*. Milton Keynes: Open University Press.

Brookfield, S. (1993) On impostership, cultural suicide, and other dangers: How nurses learn critical thinking. *The Journal of Continuing Education in Nursing* 24(5): 197-205.

Critical: at or relating to a turning point, transition or crisis; decisive: relating to criticism: rigorously discriminating: of a condition in which a chain reaction is self-sustaining.

Chambers Concise Dictionary (1985)

The philosopher Karl Popper (1970) warned us to be aware of 'the myth of the framework'. He agreed that all thought (and action) takes place within a framework - but pointed out that it is not necessary to be confined forever by it. The framework can be examined, too.

For more about this idea, see:

Barnett, R. (1994) *The Limits of Competence*. Buckingham: SRHE and Open University Press.

Popper, K. (1970) The myth of the framework. In: Lakatos, I. and Musgrave, P. (eds.) *Criticism and the Growth of Knowledge*. Cambridge: Cambridge University Press.

It is possible to use critical incident technique as a tool to examine your own practice. Generally, the technique can sharpen your awareness of underlying attitudes and assumptions.

Incidents where the outcomes are effective can highlight examples of good practice that you would like to pass on to immediate colleagues and other healthcare professionals. You could use your enquiry-based project to:

- Explore these incidents
- Put them in a theoretical framework.

Incidents where the outcomes are ineffective can reveal:

- Where you — and perhaps colleagues also — need to develop new professional skills
- Gaps in professional knowledge
- Where procedures need to be improved
- Where policies need to be reconsidered.

There is some debate about whether incidents used for critical analysis need to have made an emotional impact before they can be considered 'critical'. Flanagan, the originator of the technique, emphasises that a critical incident should be an everyday occurrence.

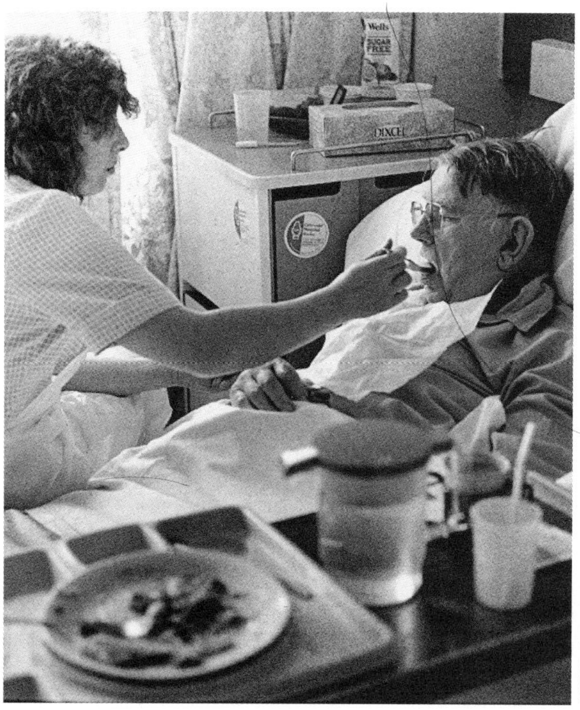

What is contained inside the moment?

What should I do?

I must answer the bell and escort the patient to the toilet

How?

I will walk with her and wait outside the toilet.

When?

As soon as I can, without putting other patients at risk.

Where?

I answer the bell wherever I am on the ward.

What happened?

Mrs M rang the bell and I went to escort her to the toilet.

What made it happen?

I had asked Mrs M to ring the bell when she needed to go to the toilet.

What does it do?

It means that I have to stop everything and go and help Mrs M

What does it feel like?

It's annoying for me sometimes, and embarrassing for Mrs M

The dialogue opposite shows how a nurse answered some of the questions in Tripp's model about the incident described on page 23.

Answer the rest of the questions in Tripp's model about the same incident.

Reflect on the situation in the photograph from the perspective of:

- The healthcare professional
- The patient.

What might a critical incident be in this case?

Clarifying the question

If you have been using the reflective and analytical techniques described in this Section, you may have at least a general idea of a topic you would like to investigate in your project. The next stage is to:

- Check that you really understand what it is you want to investigate
- Start thinking about the feasibility of your project
- Access the existing literature on the subject.

On these two pages, you will look at some fairly straightforward things you can do to clarify your question. The two following pages describe a more academic approach, using a technique called concept analysis.

Narrow the field

The issue you are interested in may be quite broad. For example, you may want to look at the way nurses interact with children who are afraid of injections. There are several issues which you could investigate here, such as:

- The range of strategies that nurses use and how effective these strategies are
- Technical innovations that could make injections less traumatic for children
- How nurses develop the skill of calming distressed children.

You might decide that your real interest is the effect of a fear of injections on patients. In this case, you could investigate:

- Children's experiences of injections
- Whether there is any relationship between adults' recollections of painful childhood injections and their attitude to the nursing profession.

There may be many aspects of an issue which interest you. You will have to decide where your priorities lie and narrow the field so your enquiry is practical and not over-ambitious.

Once you have decided where you want to focus your enquiry, define its scope more clearly. For example, the healthcare professional investigating fear of injections might need to decide:

- The setting in which the injections are given
- Whether the injections are routine inoculations or part of the treatment for a medical condition
- The age of the children.

'Forty-two!' yelled Loonquawl. 'Is that all you've got to show for seven and a half million years' work?'

'I checked it very thoroughly,' said the computer, 'and that quite definitely is the answer. I think the problem, to be quite honest with you, is that you've never actually known what the question is.'

Adams, D. (1979) *The Hitch Hiker's Guide to the Galaxy*. London: Pan.

It can be helpful to look at your independent enquiry topic from another angle. You may find that you have a stronger interest in some aspects than others. Do it in stages, like this:

- Write down your topic in the middle of a large sheet of paper
- Around it, write all the issues which you could explore
- Circle the issues which interest you most.

Ask a series of repeated questions about your topic.

I am interested in the way some healthcare professionals live such unhealthy lifestyles

Why does this matter?

Because they give health promotion information to patients and clients but ignore it themselves.

Why does this matter?

Because it undermines the message they are giving.

Why does this matter?

Because they are not acting in the best interests of patients and clients.

Why does this matter?

Because it's unprofessional.

So, what I am really interested in is whether healthcare professionals have a professional duty to maintain a healthy lifestyle.

At this point, the decision may be governed by practical considerations, such as the situation in which you work. You may also have other constraints put on you. For example, not all undergraduate researchers are encouraged to involve patients in their research.
You may have a theory that you want to test out in your project - for example, a theory that parents' attitudes to injections affect their children's behaviour. Or you may want to explore the issue without preconceptions. Both approaches are acceptable, but your decision here will have implications for the design of your research.

There is more about research design in Section 2. Section 4 shows how to finalise the wording of an enquiry question.

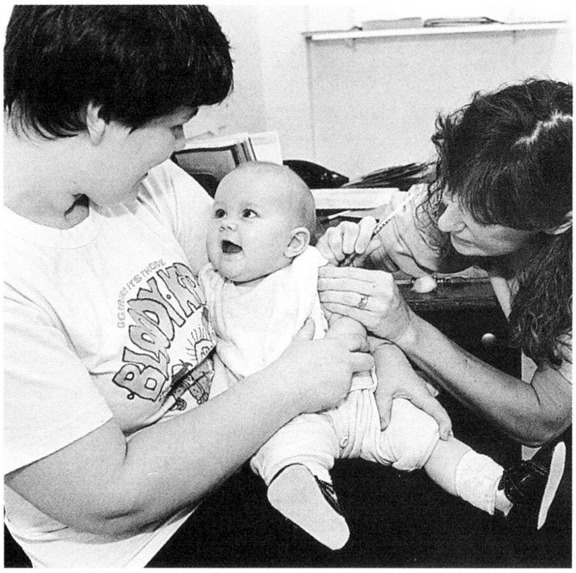
BRENDA PRINCE

A smile on her face: Trying to reassure the child

Most teachers do research for one of three purposes:

- To monitor and influence the direction of new developments
- To try to find out what is actually going on, recognising that what actually occurs is not always the same as what is thought to occur
- To evaluate what is already taking place.

Lewis, I. and Munn, P. (1987) *So you Want to Do Research? A guide for teachers on how to formulate research questions.* Edinburgh: Scottish Council for Research in Education.

Organisations define themselves by a mission statement. Write a personal mission statement for yourself. Using your personal profile to help you, complete these sentences:

My purpose as a healthcare professional is to...

As a healthcare professional, I believe that ....

My strategy to achieve my purpose is to...

Now think about your topic of enquiry. How does it contribute towards your purpose and strategy?

Think about the following questions before deciding on the topic for your project. Answer them now. If you can't, it means you need to examine your ideas more carefully.

- Am I intrinsically interested in this topic?
- What learning value does it have for me?
- How much do I already know about it?
- Are there plenty of resources on the subject?
- Can I cope with the depth and breadth needed to do it justice?
- Do the demands match the time and effort I can give it?
- Are the resources (time, facilities, money, equipment, staffing, knowledge, skills, etc.) available?
- Will I need to learn new techniques and methods?
- To whom can I go for practical help?
- Is the project open-ended or clearly-defined?
- What is likely to be the balance between practical and desk work (ie doing versus reading, collecting versus analysing) and how does this relate to my personal preferences?

(Adapted from a questionnaire for students at Oxford Brookes University.)

Analysing the concepts

In recent years, there has been a great deal of interest in defining the concepts used in the healthcare professions. Many words often found in these contexts, such as 'health' and 'care', have been used very loosely to mean a variety of different things. In an academic approach, it is essential that people involved in research and writing about these professions have a common understanding of what the terminology actually means.

Concepts

One way of defining a concept is as 'a word or term that symbolises aspects of reality that can be thought about and communicated to others.' (Waltz et al., 1991). *The Concise Oxford Dictionary* (1995) defines the word concept as 'an idea of a class of objects, or a general notion.'

Concepts can refer to things which have a physical, concrete reality, such as horses or chairs, or to abstract ideas, such as love or trust. Concepts have often been described as the building blocks for theories. If you are going to construct a theory, you need to be sure what the concepts it contains actually signify. Several authors have developed structures for analysing concepts. They follow broadly the same principles:

- Identify the concept in which you are interested
- Collect data on how it is used
- Think about a definition that covers everything you have found out about how the concept is used
- Think of a good example of the concept
- Decide how you would recognise or measure examples of the concept
- Improve your understanding by thinking of examples which might, or definitely don't, agree with your definition
- Decide if there is anything else you need to know.

A more comprehensive description of concept analysis is given opposite. The steps given here are based on a composite of several versions of the structure and are used in an article by Watson (1991) analysing the concept of 'experience'.

You will not necessarily be expected to undertake a full concept analysis for your enquiry-based project. But, you should show an awareness of how the concepts in your enquiry question are used in the literature. If you can find published concept analyses of terms you are using, they will help to clarify your thinking.

You can start to explore a concept by brainstorming all the meanings that it has for you. It is also helpful to ask your colleagues, especially those with specialist knowledge that is different from your own, for their ideas.

When you have defined your topic of enquiry, ask yourself:

- How many concepts does it contain?
- Can it be simplified so that it contains only two or three concepts?

How would you use the principles of concept analysis to explore the concept of :

- A cat
- Fear ?

Think about where you would go for your data.

- What test would you use to recognise a cat or measure fear?
- What are the critical attributes of each which fulfil the criteria for the concept?
- What examples could you could use to refine your definitions?

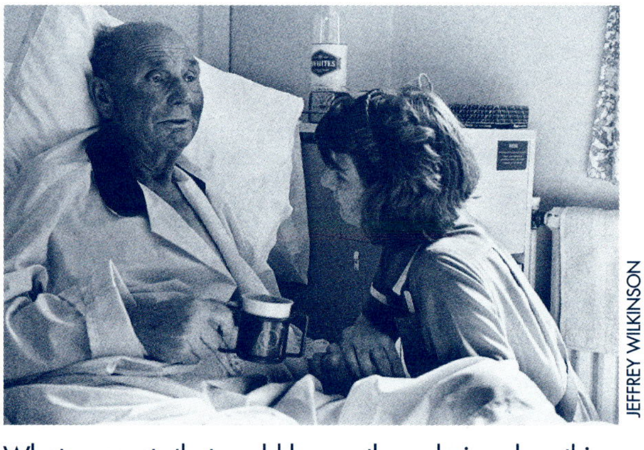

JEFFREY WILKINSON

What concepts that could be worth analysing does this photograph suggest to you?

'. . . discrete facts can be used to nail down even outrageous thoughts.'

Thomas, B. (1994) *If Monks had Macs.* New York: Voyager.

Ten steps in concept analysis

1	Identify and name the concept of interest	For example, 'experience', 'trust' or 'empowerment'.
2	Determine the aims or purpose of the study	Explain the context in which you are using a particular term and why you need to explore its meaning.
3	Identify and select an appropriate realm (sample) for data collection	Are you going to confine yourself to the literature relating directly to your profession, or will you also look in other areas?
4	Identify how the concept is used, both in everyday language, and in the particular area under study	Find examples of the term you are analysing in relevant articles and books and discuss what it is used to mean (it may involve carrying out a literature search). Also include dictionary definitions.
5	Determine the defining attributes or key areas connected with the concept. Without these attributes an example of the concept cannot occur	Think of ideas or events associated with the term. For example, one of the defining attributes of 'love' could be 'something or someone to which/whom love is directed.' In other words, you can't have love without there being an object or person to be loved.
6	Construct a model case - an example of something that unequivocally is the concept	A model case for 'experience' given in Watson (1991) is of a nurse who undergoes an intravenous pyelogram (IVP) and is subsequently better able to care for people who are themselves undergo IVP.
7	Define the empirical referents: concrete, behavioural manifestations which are required for the concept to occur, or indicate that an example of the concept has occurred	These are the things that you can measure objectively in order to decide whether or not the concept has occurred. You might test for them in an experiment or ask questions about them in an interview.
8	Construct borderline, related, contrary, invented and illegitimate examples. These help to define the limits of the concept	By thinking about situations which contradict or don't exactly fit your ideas about the concept, you can clarify what you mean. Illegitimate examples are cases where the concept is used improperly. For example, an illegitimate example of 'love' could be a mentally disturbed person who stalks and then murders the 'beloved'.
9	Identify concepts that are related to the concept of interest	These are other concepts that you might need to look at in more detail.
10	Identify areas for further study	One of the areas which Watson (1991) identified was that although 'experience' is often measured in terms of time spent doing a job, it could be more useful to find a way of measuring the 'quality' of experience in terms of the amount of learning that took place as a result of it.

An occupational therapist says:

'In my project, I wanted to look at how the previous experience of occupational therapists affected their ability to empathise with patients. I thought about what 'experience' really means - whether it can be measured by its quantity or only by its quality . Then I wrote a set of questions for my interviews with colleagues.'

'Thoughts without content are empty

Intuitions without concepts are blind.'

Kant, Immanuel. Quoted in Kolb, D. (1984) *Experiential Learning: Experience as the source of learning and development.* Englewood Cliffs, New Jersey: Prentice Hall.

If you are interested in concept analysis, you might like to look at these articles:

Meize-Grochowski, R. (1984) An analysis of the concept of trust. *Journal of Advanced Nursing* 9: 563-572.

Gibson, C.H. (1991) A concept analysis of empowerment. *Journal of Advanced Nursing* 16: 354-361.

Watson, S.J. (1991) An analysis of the concept of experience. *Journal of Advanced Nursing* 16: 1117-1121.

Recording your 'journey'

The project which you do as part of the degree programme is likely to be the most sustained piece of work you have undertaken as a student. Although you will be supported by your tutors and your colleagues, much of the responsibility for organising and carrying out the project will be down to you.

Think of an enquiry-based project as a journey. This unit will help you to prepare for the trip, but the direction you take and the experiences you have along the way cannot be predicted before you set off. Like any other traveller, you will probably make some exciting discoveries and gain interesting new perspectives. There will almost certainly be other times when you feel disheartened and disoriented.

Writing a reflective journal

If you are not already doing so, you will find it invaluable to keep a reflective journal while you are working on your project. A reflective journal is a way of recording your changing experiences and perceptions. It focuses on how events affect you and what you learn from them. It is particularly helpful when you are studying independently, as you will be when working on your project.

Your journal could contain:

- Insights
- Things that have surprised you
- Examples from your own practice, and that of others
- Difficulties and worries
- Goals
- Action plans.

You can include reflections on your studies, your professional work and everyday life. As they become absorbed in a project, many people find that the distinctions between these different areas of life become less clear cut and begin to illuminate each other. A reflective journal is an excellent way of capturing ideas and connections between ideas that might otherwise go unrecorded and be lost.

Your journal can take any form that you find helpful. Alongside your own writing, you may like to include cartoons you have cut out of the newspaper, a couple of lines from a song that capture something you are feeling, or perhaps snatches of conversation you have found relevant. You don't have to show your journal to anyone else, and the more personal it is, the more valuable it can be.

'Most of Thoreau's journal entries began as notes taken on a ramble through the woods. At the end of the day, he worked the notes into paragraphs that he then copied into blank books. When he wrote on a theme, such as moonlight, he began by pulling observations regarding the light of the moon from his journal. At first he ruined journals by ripping out the pages. Later he copied them.

The ability to structure and organise material after it is written is useful to any writer who is planning to re-use the accounts of the journal. It is also of great value to anyone trying to straighten out tangled affairs.'

Thomas, B. (1994) *If Monks had Macs*. New York: Voyager.

Students who are working independently often go through some or all of these stages:

- *Discomfiture*: expectations and assumptions are challenged, they may feel anxious and even wish to withdraw
- *Exploration*: they become more relaxed and can explore in an open and collaborative way, developing insight, confidence and satisfaction
- *Reflection and re-orientation*: they gain major insights and develop a new approach to the learning task
- *Sharing the discovery*: they test out new thinking with others
- *Equilibrium*: they elaborate, refine and apply new perspectives and approaches.

Based on Taylor, M. (1986) Learning for self-direction in the classroom: the pattern of the transition process. *Studies in Higher Education* 11(1): 55-72.

You don't have to write up a journal every night. But put aside some time every few days to keep in touch with what your topic is and how the project develops.

As well as being somewhere to collect your thoughts, a reflective journal can help you get to grips with the project in other practical ways. It can:

- Help you choose an area of practice to investigate
- Counteract feelings of isolation
- Give you a new perspective on what you are experiencing
- Prevent you from making the same mistakes twice
- Help you remember ideas you might forget
- Give you confidence that you are starting to understand and grasp the subject
- Be a storehouse of useful information
- Make you conscious of problems and stumbling blocks.

It can be very helpful to look back at your journal and add comments from a new perspective. Some people write their journal on the left hand pages of a notebook, leaving the facing pages blank for later additions.

Think about diaries and scrapbooks you may have kept in the past - perhaps to record a special event such as a holiday or the birth of a child.

- Could you use in your journal any of the techniques you used then?
- Could you try anything new?

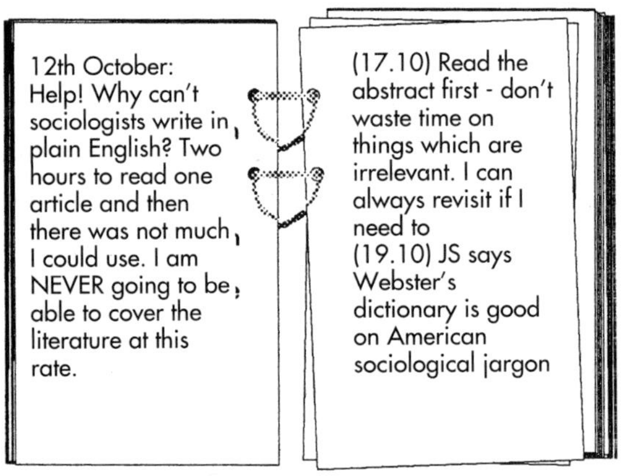

Field notes

You will probably complete your journal at a time when you can sit quietly and reflect on things. Sometimes, you will come across incidents while you are actually at work which you want to remember. Get into the habit of carrying a small notebook so that you can jot down these points. You will be able to use the notes when you write up your journal.

This is similar to the way artists make quick sketches when they are out in the field which they then work up into something more significant when they are in the studio.

If you choose an ethnographic approach in your project, you may use field notes as one of the central methods of gathering data. See Section 2 for more information about this and other approaches to research.

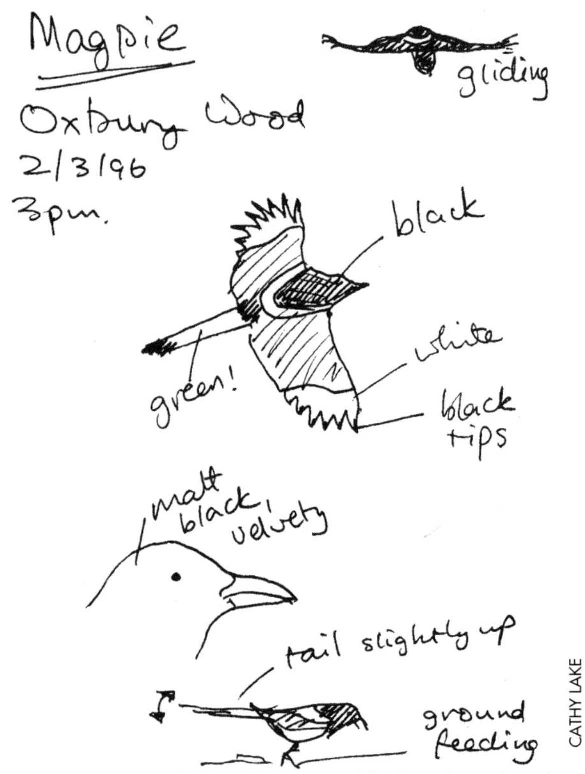

The magpie was beautiful – a matt black, velvety head and green tail. When he was flying he looked like a kite.

Conclusion

The reflective and analytical techniques described in this first Section should help you develop the habit of questioning your actions and assumptions. Their aim is to:

- Encourage you to look at your work from new perspectives
- Help you recognise issues to be explored in more detail
- Start you thinking about the topic and the scope of your enquiry-based project.

A good project should result in new knowledge which adds to the understanding of the researcher and other healthcare professionals. By now you may be able to identify an area of work where you want to increase your understanding and knowledge. You should be choosing a topic which is closely related to your own interests, values and priorities and which you are strongly motivated to investigate.

At this stage, you may not have formalised the exact wording of your research question. That can come later, when you have found out more about the implications of different types of research design and started to plan your project in detail. But you should already be aware of the importance of limiting the scope of your enquiries to a manageable size and of clarifying the concepts you are looking at.

Inevitably, your plans will change as you work through the enquiry. But if you start with a clear idea of what you want to investigate, it will be much easier to decide on appropriate methods for your study.

> 'But it was the Great Question! The Ultimate Question of Life, the Universe and Everything,' howled Loonquawl.
>
> 'Yes', said Deep Thought with the air of one who suffers fools gladly, 'but what actually is it?'...
>
> 'Well, you know, it's just Everything... Everything...' offered Phouchg weakly.
>
> 'Exactly!' said Deep Thought. 'So once you do know what the question actually is, you'll know what the answer means.'
>
> Adams, D. (1979) *The Hitch Hiker's Guide to the Galaxy*. London: Pan.

References

Boud D., Keogh R. and Walker D. (1985) *Reflection: Turning experience into learning.* London: Kogan Page.

Carper, B. (1978) Fundamental patterns of knowing in nursing. *Advances in Nursing Science* 1: 13-23.

Flanagan, J. C. (1954) The critical incident technique. *Psychological Bulletin* 5: 327-358.

Johns, C. (1994) Nuances of reflection. *Journal of Clinical Nursing* 3: 71-75.

Mezirow, J. (1981) A critical theory of adult learning and eduction. *Adult Eduction* 32 (1): 3–24.

Tripp, D. (1993) *Critical Incidents in Teaching.* London: Routledge.

Waltz, C., Strickland, O. and Lenz, E. (1991) *Measurement in Nursing Research.* Philadelphia: F.A. Davis Company.

Watson, S. J. (1991) An analysis of the concept of experience. *Journal of Advanced Nursing* 16: 1117-1121.

Introduction

This Section explores what is meant by the terms 'research' and 'enquiry' and how they differ from other methods of finding things out.

There are several approaches to research or enquiry, ranging from the classic laboratory experiment in which objectivity must be maintained at all costs, to the method known as 'action research', in which the researcher works to solve a problem at the same time as doing the study.

The Section also introduces various paradigms for enquiry into practice and explains the different perspectives and philosophies on which they are based. It will help you to:

- Become familiar with a range of approaches to enquiry
- Decide which of them is most appropriate for your own project.

Follow up your study of the Section by reading some of the recommended texts which discuss the theory of research in more detail.

In the context of professional work, enquiry and research are much the same thing. There is no need to see the research process as something very different from what you do normally. It is much more important to be concerned that the enquiry you are carrying out is done properly, so that you and others can learn from the outcomes.

Although the enquiry should be independent, this does not mean you have to do it in isolation. If the topic of enquiry relates closely to your work, other people around you will be important collaborators in the research. You may be talking to them about it, getting their help, asking them what they think about your findings. In some cases, your enquiry may be part of a piece of research on a larger scale involving several independent enquiries.

You may be looking at an issue from one point of view, while others are looking at it from different points. In the social sciences, 'multi-method' research is seen as providing valuable insights into the real world, and usually cannot be described or interpreted fully by a single researcher, no matter how thorough the enquiry.

'It is, in fact, nothing short of a miracle that the modern methods of instruction have not yet entirely strangled the holy curiosity of inquiry; for this delicate little plant, aside from stimulation, stands mainly in need of freedom; without this it goes to wrack and ruin without fail.'

Albert Einstein, quoted in Rogers, C. (1983) *Freedom to Learn for the 80s*. New York: Macmillan.

'I have found that "research" tends to put some people off. They see it as some esoteric enterprise necessarily done by outside experts. In fact, it is simply another word for 'enquiry'...'

Robson, C. (1993) *Real World Research: A resource for social scientists and practitioner-researchers*. Oxford: Blackwell.

Here are some of the words used in this Section. As you come across them you might like to:

- Look them up in a dictionary
- Think about their meanings in relation to research
- Write down in your learning journal how they relate to your practice.

Deductive	Positivism
Inductive	Ethic
Quantitative	Phenomenon
Qualitative	Emancipatory
Paradigm	

How do you find out things?

The skills needed to be a researcher are not so very different from the skills used in everyday life when you want to find out things.

Suppose you wanted to find out about taking a holiday in a country you had never visited. In this situation, you might:

- Talk to friends who had been there
- Talk to someone who lives there
- Get advice from a travel agent
- Read books and magazine articles about the country
- Watch TV dramas and documentaries set in the country
- Read technical information in brochures about booking a holiday.

You probably wouldn't take everything you were told at face value, but would interpret the information you gathered. For example, you might discount the views of a particular individual if you knew her tastes were very different from your own.

If you were planning to go on holiday with someone else, you might summarise what you have found out and report your conclusions to the individual.

All these activities have their parallels in the process of enquiring into practice. When you choose a holiday you are, in effect:

- Asking questions
- Collecting and analysing data
- Interpreting the evidence, coming to a conclusion and reporting on your findings.

But there are significant differences between the kind of enquiry you make in ordinary life and the way you conduct an enquiry-based project.

Polit and Hungler (1993) identified five different sources of knowledge that people frequently use to make decisions:

- Tradition
- Authorities
- Human experience
- Trial and error
- Logical reasoning.

For example, when making a decision about a holiday destination, some people's thinking might go along one of these lines:

- 'We always go to Spain.'
- 'The travel agent said that this company gave the best deal.'
- 'I always enjoy sailing holidays.'

Look at the following methods of acquiring information used in everyday life.

- Directories
- The Internet
- Talking to experts
- Talking to friends and colleagues
- Books
- Magazines
- TV programmes
- Catalogues
- CD-ROM.

With which methods do you feel most comfortable?

Which do you find most reliable?

Your answers may have implications for the enquiry methods you select later.

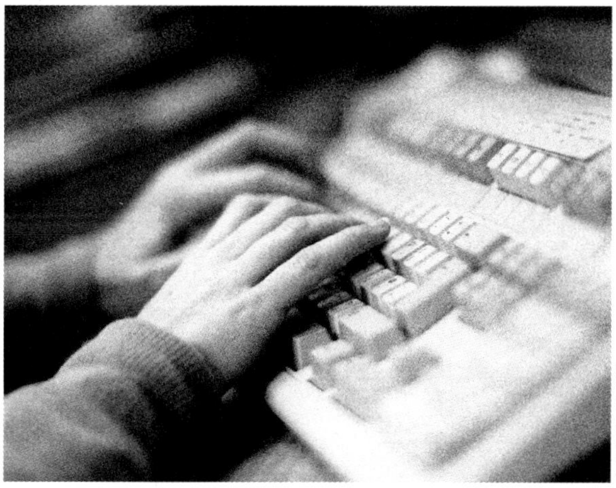

RICHARD SMITH

What methods of acquiring information has information technology opened up for you at work?

If you are interested in information technology, see the unit entitled *Health Care and the Information Age*.

- 'France was awful last year, so this year we'll try Portugal.'
- 'I don't want to go anywhere too hot. Scandinavia has good temperatures at this time of year.'

All these methods have their drawbacks. If you are guided solely by what you are familiar with, you will miss out on new experiences; experts can give incomplete or partial advice; trial and error can lead to a succession of disasters; logical reasoning is only as good as the completeness and accuracy of the information on which you base your argument.

Enquiry into practice involves a systematic approach to gathering and evaluating information. It is concerned with building new knowledge and understanding, not with uncritically adopting established opinions.

The approach has more in common with the kind of investigations you make when you are exploring a subject in which you have a genuine personal interest. In these cases, you usually welcome new perspectives and insights. You are willing to compare and contrast them with your own knowledge and experience.

The approach you adopt in enquiry should be both systematic and critical. When you conduct a piece of research, you become an 'expert' in a particular, limited field, even if your expertise extends only to an accurate understanding of the limitations of your present knowledge.

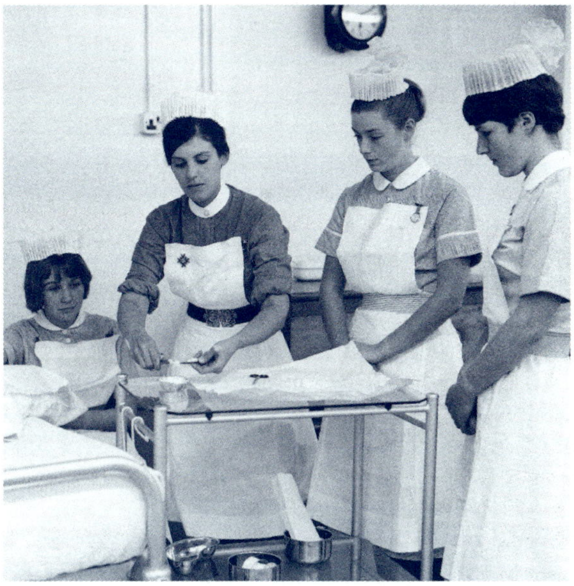

NURSING TIMES

A traditional ward scene from around 20 years ago

Healthcare professionals are sometimes criticised for an over-reliance on logical reasoning:

'When French women started to complain that their supposedly "painless childbirth" as the Lamaze method is referred to in France, had actually been for some of them unbearably painful, one French obstetrician wrote in *Le Monde* that it was impossible that a woman well prepared in the Lamaze technique could suffer pain and that no painkillers or anaesthesia were needed. If a woman did suffer, he said, it was because she had started her training too late or had not worked at it hard enough, or that the obstetrical team had not taken the method seriously.'

Payer, L. (1990) *Medicine and Culture: Notions of health and sickness*. London: Victor Gollancz.

Think of times, at work or at home, when you have made decisions in any of the ways described above by Polit and Hungler. What was the effect?

How did the limitations of knowledge of healthcare professionals 20 years ago affect the way they worked?

Imagine someone in 20 years time looking at a photograph taken today of healthcare professionals at work. What might they say about the limitations of our present knowledge?

What are the limitations of present knowledge in the area you have chosen for your enquiry?

'We shall not cease from exploration
And the end of all exploring
Will be to arrive where we started
And know the place for the first time.'

Eliot, T. S. (1995) *The Four Quartets*. London: Faber.

Methods of enquiry used in health care

As a healthcare professional, you participate routinely in several different forms of information-gathering. Many of the techniques will be similar to those you could use in your project.

Care planning

In your work with people, you collect information about their needs and monitor how these needs are being met. The usual way to do this is to fill in a type of questionnaire while interviewing the patient/client. You will also observe the person, noticing and recording significant changes in behaviour and take measurements such as pulse and temperature.

These are all techniques which could be used in a project, but in the context of everyday health care they have a different purpose. In day-to-day work, they are used purely for the benefit of the patient or client under consideration. In an enquiry-based project, they could be used to improve care for other patients or to extend the researcher's knowledge in other ways.

Audit

An audit is a methodical review. Audit has become an important part of life in the health services in recent years because of the need to ensure and demonstrate that resources are being used in the most effective way, and that the quality standards laid down in contracts are being maintained. Many professionals have approached audit by another route, from an interest in quality management methodology, such as quality circles, total quality management (TQM) and standard-setting.

There are six areas to be considered when undertaking audit, working outwards from direct involvement with the patient:

- Clinical care
- Workload management
- Deployment
- Personnel management
- Organisational arrangements
- Environment and support.

Your own enquiry could deal with any of these six areas.

Ethically, it is important that patients consent to their participation in research and understand the difference between the role of the health-care professional as researcher and carer.

- Do you find that patients object to answering questions if they feel it will help you provide the best possible care for them?
- What reaction do you think patients would have if they suspected you were asking questions for another purpose?
- How could it affect your relationship?
- What methods of gathering and evaluating data do you use at each stage of the care planning cycle?

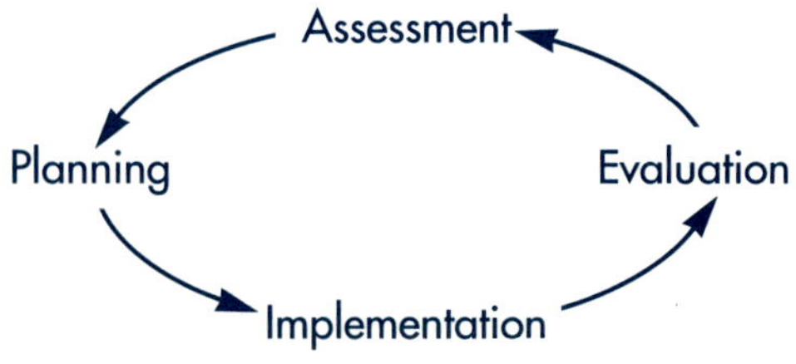

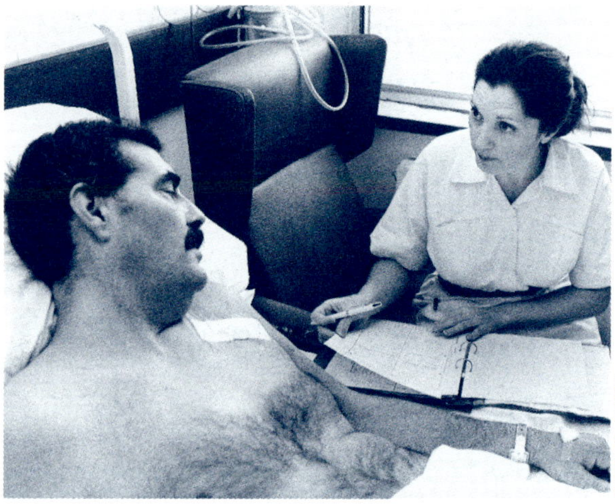

Assessing, planning, implementing or evaluating?

The unit *Professional Relationships: Influences on health care* considers in more depth the way you can affect relationships with colleagues and clients. The unit *Healthcare Evaluation* looks in some detail at interview techniques.

Once the decision about which area to audit has been made, there are four stages to the audit process:

- Objective-/standard-setting
- Implementation
- Measuring and recording
- Monitoring and action plan.

The Framework document (see below) lists several methods of audit which are in widespread use in health care:

- Peer review
- Questionnaires (patient- and staff-based)
- Sample surveys
- Direct observation of staff and/or patients — organisation and management (O&M) studies
- Self-recording by staff of what is done
- Statistical evaluation against pre-defined formulae/standards
- Spot checks, for example on data/records
- Trend analyses
- Comparative analyses.

Any experience you have had with auditing tools can help if your project uses any of these techniques. But remember that, in your own enquiry, you will be collecting and evaluating information for a purpose other than audit. In particular, audit looks at specific examples of what has been done, or is being done, and checks how they measure against pre-set criteria. It does not seek to find new knowledge or to set things in a wider, theoretical context.

Some quality initiatives are closer to the spirit of practice-based enquiry as they may involve participants in conducting research. An example is quality circles, in which professionals sit down and discuss questions such as 'Is there a better way that we could be doing this?' Even so, within the constraints of working for an organisation, solutions are likely to be locally based and may not reflect the full range of possibilities described in the literature. Your research project provides an opportunity to explore these possibilities in more depth.

'Nursing audit is part of the cycle of quality assurance. It incorporates the systematic and critical analyses by nurses, midwives and health visitors, in conjunction with other staff, of the planning, delivery and evaluation of nursing and midwifery care, in terms of their use of resources and the outcomes for patients/clients, and introduces appropriate change in response to that analysis.'

Definition of nursing audit by Project 32, quoted in: NHS Management Executive (1991) *Framework of Audit for Nursing Services*. London: NHS Management Executive.

'I am a member of a quality group within my unit looking at the results of a recent restructuring. I had already established a good rapport with the other members of staff. I saw my project as an opportunity to try out a piece of practical action research with them, focusing on clinical flexibility.'

Jane, a physiotherapist

The unit *Healthcare Evaluation* looks in more detail at the audit process as part of evaluation.

Here are four audit tools used for nursing:

- Dynamic Standard Setting System (DySSy) produced by the RCN
- Phaneuf's Nursing Audit, based on a retrospective audit of care plans
- Monitor, based on the American Rush Medicus system, which combines an analysis of chart information with observation of nursing care
- Qualpacs, in which trained assessors evaluate care against certain criteria.

Which of these audit methods do you find yields the most useful information:

- For you as a professional?
- For the organisation for which you work?

Which method (or methods) do you think most appropriate to your own approach to patient care?

What is enquiry?

To enquire is to seek information about, to question or to investigate. Enquiry into an aspect of your own practice is a form of research: 'careful search or inquiry; endeavour to discover new facts by scientific study' (*Concise Oxford Dictionary*, 1995). Research and enquiry are part of the same process.

The process of academic enquiry is summarised on the opposite page. Academic enquiry has these four defining characteristics:

- It is a process by which information is gathered and evaluated and is made conscious and explicit
- Results are made accessible to other people
- It involves the development of new knowledge
- It sets new knowledge in the context of what is already known about the process.

The systematic nature of the enquiry method sets it apart from the more casual enquiries made in everyday life, and from investigations in working life where theories are applied to a particular situation but may not be tested or challenged.

The four characteristics of academic enquiry have two main advantages. First, they give a framework around which to organise the project. It isn't necessary to reinvent the wheel every time a new project begins. As later pages in this Section show, there are actually many frameworks, or paradigms, around which an enquiry-based project can be designed.

Second, because enquiry follows established rules, it is easier for other people to learn from previous studies. Policy-makers can also have confidence in conclusions drawn from a properly conducted study.

The main drawback of the academic process, from the point of view of the enquirer, is that it demands an understanding of technical concepts and methodology which may seem to have little to do directly with professional interests. Some enquiry methods, particularly those involving complex statistical analysis, require specialised knowledge. But many other methods are much more accessible. If you get into the habit of reading research reports, you will probably find that most of them are less daunting than you first thought, once you have got through the initial language barrier.

On this page and the next are several definitions of research and enquiry. Before you read them, write your own definition of practice-based enquiry.

'Research seeks answers to questions in an orderly and systematic way. It is a method of problem-solving - just as the nursing process is a method of organising the delivery of nursing care in clinical practice. The answers to nursing research questions help nurses to provide more effective nursing care and to document the unique role nursing plays in the healthcare system. Nursing research extends the base of information not only for the nurse asking the question but also for other nurses seeking answers to the same problem.'

Polit, D.F. and Hungler, B.P. (1993) *Essentials of Nursing Research* (3rd edition). Philadelphia: J.B. Lippincott Company.

'The systematic, controlled, empirical and critical investigation of hypothetical propositions and the presumed relations among natural phenomena.'

Kerlinger, F. N. (1970) *Foundations of Behavioural Research*. London: Holt Rinehart & Winston.

'Any systematic and rigorous inquiry which seeks to describe, explain, measure, challenge, further elucidate, test or theorise about some activity, process or phenomena.'

Davis, P. (1992) *Supervision*. Unpublished seminar paper in a series presented in Oxford at the National Institute of Nursing

Ask your colleagues in the multidisciplinary team for their definitions of enquiry or research.

In what way do they differ from your own?

The process of academic enquiry

Conceptual phase Developing the design	• Defining the problem - what will be studied • Literature review • Statement of purpose - the rationale for the study and its focus • Selecting the research design • Specifying the population sample • Developing a plan for data collection • Identifying the limitations.
Empirical phase Data collection	• Formulation of data collection instruments, ie questionnaire, interview schedule, observation schedule, experiment, etc. • Data collection activity.
Interpretative phase Analysing and interpreting the data	• Data analysis • Interpreting the results - is there sufficient evidence in the data to support the hypothesis or to answer the research question? - what else needs to be done or what other questions need to be asked? - what conclusions can be drawn and what do they mean? • Writing and communicating the results of the study.

'Research in its broadest sense is an attempt to gain solutions to problems. More precisely, it is the collection of data in a rigorously controlled situation for the purpose of prediction or explanation.'

Treece, E. and Treece, J. (1986) *Elements of Research in Nursing* (4th edition) St Louis: C.V. Mosby Company.

'An attempt to increase the sum of what is known, usually referred to as a "body of knowledge", by discovery of new facts or relationships through a process of systematic scientific enquiry, the research process.'

Macleod Clark, J. and Hockey, L. (1989) *Further Research for Nursing*. London: Scutari Press.

Look through the summary above of the enquiry process.

- Which parts of it do you feel you already know something about?
- Which parts do you think will be most challenging to you?

Record your reactions in your reflective journal. You might like to return to them later, when you are working on your project.

Enquiring into practice

Research and enquiry are happening all the time in health care. However, it is only in the past 25 years that it has been thought necessary that all healthcare professionals have an understanding of the practice of research (Hopps, 1994). The volume of research has grown considerably in this time as the academic and professional stature of the professions has developed.

Nursing

Florence Nightingale wrote about the importance of research in nursing, but very little work was done for about a century. The first studies in the UK were undertaken by sociologists and psychologists but at the end of the 1950s Marjorie Simpson set up a self-help group for nurse researchers known as the Research Discussion Group.

In the 1960s the Department of Health and Social Security (DHSS) funded a research project, *The Study of Nursing Care*, to establish how to measure the quality of nursing care. The 14 studies in this project (summarised by Inman (1975), mark the beginning of modern research into nursing problems by nurses themselves.

Interest in nursing research grew in the 1970s, with the recommendation in the Briggs report that nursing should become 'a research-based profession' (DHSS, 1972(a)). As a result, the appreciation of research became part of nurse training at basic and post-basic levels. The White Paper *A Framework for Government Research and Development* (DHSS 1972(b)) led to the setting up of the Nursing Research Liaison Officer Scheme, which made links between research, practice and education.

The Report of the Royal Commission on the National Health Service (1979) identified several key areas for research, including standards of care, primary health care and the need to define clinical roles. Research in other areas began, as well:

- In 1983, national workshops for senior nurse managers were set up to explore how research could be made a priority at health authority level
- In 1991 the ENB described a five-year research and development plan in its annual report
- In 1993 the *Report of the Taskforce on a Strategy for Research in Nursing, Midwifery and Health Visiting* announced a co-ordinated strategy for research in nursing as a whole (DoH, 1993[a]).

Find out if any of the initiatives described on these two pages have had any influence on your local health authority.

- What research has been done in recent years?
- Has it resulted in changes in policy or practice?
- What research is currently under way?
- Is there any way in which you feel you could contribute to this research yourself?

'Research is... not a luxury for the academic, but a tool for developing the quality of nursing decisions, prescriptions and actions. Whether as clinicians, educators, managers or researchers we have a research responsibility: neglect of that responsibility could be classed as professional negligence.'

Clamp, C.G.L. (1991) *Resources for Nursing Research: An annotated bibliography*. London: Library Association Publishing.

Get hold of the academic journals which apply to your own professional group. Look out for articles related to your enquiry topic. What are the main issues being researched at the moment?

You could log them in your reflective journal or include them in your personal profile – and note how the issues change over time.

'Nursing research is defined as research into those aspects of professional activity which are predominantly and appropriately the concerns and responsibilities of nurses.'

Cormack, D. (1991) *The Research Process in Nursing*. Oxford: Blackwell.

Chapman (1996) notes that 'the amount of nursing research has increased in recent years...a considerable amount of research... comes from abroad... all these small contributions to nursing knowledge need to be combined and compared if nurses are to be able to evaluate the findings and apply them appropriately to practice.'

Occupational therapy and physiotherapy

A similar picture of development through three decades can be drawn for occupational therapy. A firm scientific base for the profession started to be built during the 1960s. Until then, the theoretical base was 'embryonic' and there were no 'systematic statements regarding...the nature of physical and psychological change processes' (Mosey, 1971). During the 1960s and 1970s, professionals in the field began to put together a core of knowledge about 'occupation' and its relationship to health and well-being (Christiansen, 1991).

In the 1980s the new discipline of occupational science - defined as 'the systematic study of humans as occupational beings' – emerged to support therapeutic practice. Research studies carried out during the decade showed that 'engagement in ...ordinary daily activities (that is, occupations) significantly affects health, happiness and life satisfaction' (Carlson and Clark, 1991). By the 1990s the idea that occupational therapists should be actively involved in research as a normal part of their work was widely accepted.

A similar position has been taken by physiotherapists, where 'the critical stance of a reflective practitioner' is seen to be relevant throughout the profession (Richardson, 1993). Research is needed in order to create and sustain a body of practice-based knowledge.

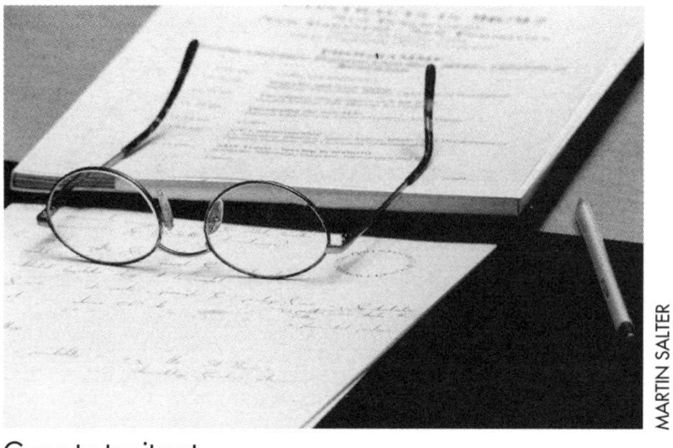
MARTIN SALTER

Gone to try it out

'An important function of occupational science is to provide basic knowledge that supports the applied practice of occupational therapy.'

Yerxa, E., Clark, F., Frank, G. et al. (1989) An introduction to occupational science: A foundation for occupational therapy in the 21st century. *Occupational Therapy in Health Care* 6(4): 1-17.

'Experiment and observation are particularly applicable in occupational therapy, where the outcome of much of the therapist's work is based upon the act of looking, the art of observation and the application of imagination.' Goble, R. (1989) Research in occupational therapy: luxury or necessity? *British Journal of Occupational Therapy* 52(9): 349-51.

'...the changes now in health care suggest that education and research should be led by practice in order to identify the new competences and strategies being developed and used successfully in practice today. ...Along with changes in the patterns of employment and deployment of physiotherapists this suggests that recently qualified and inexperienced staff will have to become independent, autonomous professionals without the luxury of being able to follow set paths of practice or to work closely with senior staff.'

Richardson, B. (1993) Practice, research and education - what is the link? *Physiotherapy* 79(5): 317-22.

How can carrying out research help to create healthcare practitioners who are able to deal effectively with the healthcare needs of the 1990s and beyond?

How useful is research?

The ultimate purpose of research in health care must be to improve practice. In order to obtain funding from the NHS, a research project has to demonstrate that it will be of practical value to other professionals and that it will contribute to increasing the effectiveness of services.

It is easy to see the practical use of some studies. For example, an enquiry-based project which compares waiting times and procedures in two clinics could result in immediate increases in efficiency.

Some of the more theoretical areas of research are more difficult to justify in practical terms. For example, what benefits result from a study of the language people use to describe depression? One answer is that theoretical work of this kind can lay the foundations for other studies with very practical applications.

In relatively new academic disciplines, such as nursing and other professions allied to medicine, it is sometimes necessary to clarify the conceptual framework before proceeding to more practical studies.

The Health of the Nation report (DoH, 1991) states that 'Research is essential to any strategy to improve health'. At the same time as the overall research strategy was being developed, a separate taskforce was set up in 1992 to advise on a strategy for research in nursing, midwifery and health visiting and the strategy was launched in 1993 (DoH, 1993(a)). Its recommendations aim 'to integrate research by the nursing professions and research into nursing issues within the R&D strategy....the broad thrust of the recommendations also have relevance to physiotherapy, occupational therapy and speech and language therapy.'

In 1993 the Department of Health published details of its research and development strategy (DoH, 1993[b]). The strategy affirms that research is an integral component of health and social care policy, management, patient care and the delivery of social services.

An important feature of the strategy is that it will closely involve NHS staff. Their role will be to:

- Identify important issues and characterise and prioritise these problems as the basis for seeking solutions

'When the neutron was first found, its study amounted to research of the purest kind. Nobody could have foreseen any practical use for it. This changed dramatically with the discovery (1939) that neutrons could cause the fission of uranium nuclei, with the liberation of more neutrons; in this way a chain reaction became possible, and this is now our chief source of neutrons and an increasingly important source of power. Today neutrons are an industrial commodity; several tons have been produced (and immediately consumed) in the brief history of atomic energy. Only ten years elapsed between the discovery of the neutron and the operation of the first atomic pile!'

Otto Frisch explains atomic particles; quoted in Carey, J. (1995) *The Faber Book of Science*. London: Faber and Faber Ltd.

A useful book which looks at the main themes of nursing practice, care delivery, research training and career development is:

Fitzpatrick, J.J., Stevenson, J.S. and Polis, N.S. (1995) *Nursing Research and its Utilization*. New York: Springer Publishing Co.

Look at the criteria listed above for research and development from the NHS Research and Development Task Force.

- Can you see why an audit would not meet these criteria?
- It is not essential that your own project meets these criteria, but do you think it should?
- If your project does not meet the criteria, do you consider it in anyway less valuable?

If you are thinking of applying for a grant, you might find it useful to look at *The Grant Application Writers' Handbook* by L. Reif-Lehrer, (1995). London: Jones and Bartlett.

- Help to set the agenda for research
- Carry out applied research, especially in multidisciplinary teams
- Ensure that practice reflects research-based knowledge.

To support the strategy, programmes have been set up to identify research issues in particular areas such as diseases, health technologies and client groups. Regional plans have also been set up in the 14 regions and networks are developing to support researchers and help disseminate the results. A register of research projects is kept at a regional level and these are assembled into a national database.

A report to the Minister for Health by a research and development task force chaired by Professor Anthony Culyer (NHS Research and Development Task Force, 1994), recommended that all research and development whose direct costs are met with NHS funds should:

- Be designed to provide new knowledge needed to improve the performance of the NHS in improving the health of the nation
- Be designed so that findings will be of value to those in the NHS facing similar problems outside the particular locality or context of the project, that is, be generalisable
- Follow a clear, well-defined protocol
- Have had the protocol reviewed by peers
- Have obtained the approval, where needed, of the local research ethics committee and any other appropriate body
- Have clearly defined arrangements for the findings of project management plans to be reported so that they are open to critical examination and accessible to all who could benefit from them; this will normally involve publication.

'Research is stimulating. It does not have to be something done in an ivory tower by being remote from clinical practice. It can be a fully routine part of clinical practice, benefiting the patient and the clinician alike. The patient benefits from maximum clinical effectiveness; the clinician by involvement in an absorbing process that becomes endless and addictive. Answering one question leads to asking another, which leads to... Try it.'

Brooks, N. (1988) Why research? *British Journal of Occupational Therapy* 51(11): 397-98.

'Nursing is dynamic and interactive and it could be suggested that the rigorous academic approach to scientific research cannot appropriately integrate nursing theory and practice. A more reflexive approach involving a participative and collaborative style of research to bridge the theory/practice gap might be appropriate both for nursing and other professionals using practical skills.'

Green, S. (1991) Weaving the web of knowledge. *The Health Service Journal* 101 (September 19): 22-23.

What impact is the DoH research and development strategy (DoH 1993(b)) having on your area of practice? Find out:

- The research priorities for your region (stated in the regional plan)
- How research results are communicated to healthcare professionals
- What networks have developed to support research and the dissemination of results.

Think about how your enquiry topic might fit in or relate to the regional plan.

Quantitative and qualitative research

There are two main branches of research. Quantitative research is concerned with measuring things against pre-set criteria. Qualitative research attempts to explore the characteristics of things without preconceptions. The two branches reflect different views of the world and imply different relationships between the researcher and the researched.

Quantitative research

In natural sciences such as chemistry and biology, the objectivity of the researcher is seen to be crucial. Research is carefully designed to eliminate bias or contamination. Researchers start by formulating a hypothesis which they test out in experiments, surveys or trials, using large numbers of subjects to reduce the effects of maverick results.

In quantitative research, researchers are looking for answers to pre-set questions. They are seeking to impose a framework of rules or ideas on the data they have collected. The idea which underpins quantitative research is that results obtained can be generalised across a wider population than the sample which was studied.

Qualitative research

Social or human scientists believe that reality is variable, depending on the experiences of the individual. Although the results of research may hold meaning for other individuals and society, they cannot be applied generally. It is a central tenet of the qualitative approach that the researcher inevitably affects the knowledge generated in several ways - including the questions that are asked, the choice of methods for collection, and the processing and presentation of results - and that this effect should be acknowledged.

Much social science research is concerned with human behaviour and the relationships that individuals or groups of people have with their surroundings and each other. The research activity often takes place in natural settings, such as the work environment, rather than the laboratory or the carefully controlled sample groups used in quantitative research. The data from such studies cannot all be quantified but are dependent on the quality of the representations of human existence under study.

In quantitative research, you look at the world as an observer. In qualitative research, you try to get inside the world you are observing.

There is an interesting discussion of quantitative and qualitative research in nursing in:

Duffy, M. E. (1985) Designing nursing research: the qualitative-quantitative debate. *Journal of Advanced Nursing* 10: 225-232.

Which approach would be more useful if you wanted to find out:

- Whether there was a relationship between what a patient was told about pain control before a surgical operation and the level of pain control necessary afterwards?
- The language patients used to describe post-operative pain?

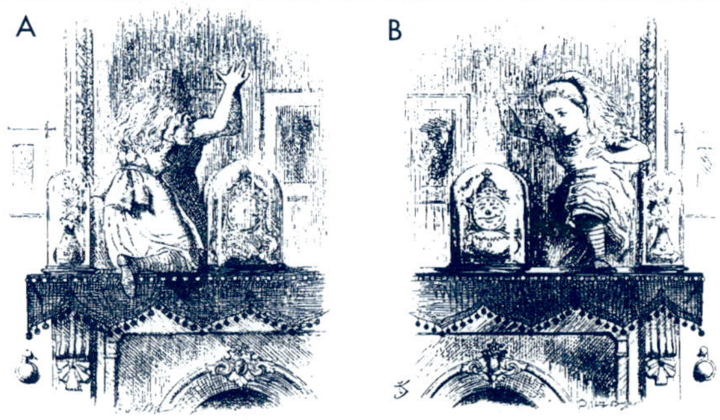

MACMILLAN

A: 'It's very like our passage as far as I can see, only, you know, it may be quite different beyond.'

B: '... such beautiful things in it. Let's pretend there's a way of getting through into it, somehow, Kitty.'

Alice Through the Looking Glass — Lewis Carroll.

'I wouldn't trust that computer to speak my weight,' said Ford.

'I can do that for you, sure,' enthused the computer punching out more tickertape. 'I can even work out your personality problems to ten decimal places if it will help.'

Adams, D. (1979) *The Hitch Hiker's Guide to the Galaxy*. London: Pan.

Deductive and inductive reasoning

Deductive reasoning uses general rules to make predictions about specific situations. It builds on previous knowledge to construct theories which can be tested by experiment. Deductive reasoning is used in clinical research. For example, if a researcher knows that a particular drug has a beneficial effect on a certain medical condition, an experiment could be designed to find out whether a related drug had similar effects. Deductive reasoning forms the basis for quantitative research.

Inductive reasoning moves from the specific to the general. The researcher describes a situation, looking for patterns and relationships. These are then used to identify concepts and develop a theory about what is happening. Inductive reasoning is commonly used in qualitative research.

Deductive reasoning is appropriate when the researcher wishes to test a theory. Inductive reasoning is more appropriate if the researcher is not sure what is going on, or suspects that the situation may be more complex than existing theories allow for.

Researchers often use both deductive and inductive reasoning in their research. They might start by looking at a situation inductively to establish what appears to be happening. Then they construct a theory which they test out with deductive reasoning.

For example, a researcher might carry out a study to discover the opinions of people who had recently attended a particular clinic. Her data might reveal that many of the people expressed dissatisfaction that they were not seen in person by the consultant. This knowledge could be reached inductively, by looking for patterns in the interviews. The researcher could then develop a theory that there was a relationship between patients' level of satisfaction with their treatment and whether they were seen by the consultant or a less senior member of staff. The theory could be tested by looking at the data again in the light of it, or designing a survey to find out if this theory was more generally applicable.

Quantitative	Qualitative
• Reality is singular	• Realities are multiple, interrelated
• Objective reality comprises the domain of science	• Subjective experiences are as legitimate as objective information
• The appropriate approach to discovering reality is reductionistic	• An ecological approach provides a full understanding of reality
• Through knowledge of the parts, knowledge of the whole can be accumulated	• The whole is greater than the sum of the parts
• Discrepancies in data must be accounted for or eliminated	• Discrepancies may be existentially real

From Haase, J. E. and Myers, S. T. (1988) Reconciling paradigm assumptions of qualitative and quantitative research. *Western Journal of Nursing Research* 10(2): 128-137.

There is a fascinating discussion of the differences between the quantitative and qualitative approaches, and ways in which they can work together, in:

Bryman, A. (1988) *Quantity and Quality in Social Research*. London: Routledge.

For insight into the theoretical basis of scientific research, see:

Chambers, A.F. (1978) *What is This Thing Called Science?* Milton Keynes: Open University Press.

Wider issues related to social research methods, such as the need to consider theories, assumptions and philosophical perspectives which underpin these issues, are looked at in:

Davidson, J. O. and Layder, D. (1995) *Methods, Sex and Madness*. London: Routledge.

How could deductive and inductive reasoning be used to investigate a situation where a particular primary or secondary care unit has an extremely high turnover of staff?

Research paradigms — 1

Quantitative and qualitative approaches can be further divided into several distinct research paradigms. A research paradigm is a model with its own methods and world view. These models can be arranged along a continuum, as in the diagram below. At the left-hand end of the scale is the positivist model, where the objectivity of the researcher is paramount. The aim of this type of research is to discover how existing rules apply in a particular situation. It is the classic quantitative approach.

As you move further along the scale, more importance is given to understanding a situation from the point of view of its participants:

- Ethnography is concerned with developing theories from close study of how individuals and groups interact in particular situations
- Phenomenology does not attempt to develop theories. Its task is to describe accurately the experience of living through the situation
- Emancipatory research takes on a practical and even political role. The aim is to empower individuals to examine and improve their own practice.

The positivist approach to enquiry is based on the belief that reality is constant and that knowledge gained in one situation can be applied in another situation. Within positivism, the two most widely used methods of obtaining information are through experiments and surveys.

Experiments

An experiment is an attempt to control reality so that researchers can see the effect of changing particular aspects of it. For example, different drugs are tried out on a group of volunteers. The validity of the experiment will depend to a large extent on whether the researchers can show that all other conditions are identical. If the only variable was the nature of the drug given to the volunteers, any differences in the way they respond can be attributed to the effects of the drug. But this is not as easy as it seems. Even under laboratory conditions, it can be difficult to eliminate all other variables. When researchers are studying human behaviour, rather than clinical symptoms, the difficulties can become insurmountable.

The first stage in designing an experiment is to write a hypothesis. This usually suggests a causal relationship between two variables, such as the time spent talking to patients on admission to hospital and the degree of satisfaction with their

Quantitative			Qualitative
Positivism	Ethnography	Phenomenology	Emancipatory research

The continuum presents a very simplified picture of the relationship between research paradigms. As you read more about the different approaches, you may find it helpful to produce a more complex model of your own.

'It is a wise experimenter who knows his artefact from his main effect and wiser still is the researcher who realises that today's artefact may be tomorrow's independent variable.'

McGuire, W. J. (1969) Suspiciousness of experimenters' intent. In: Rosenthal, R. and Rosnow, R. L. (eds.) *Artefact in Behavioural Research*. New York: Academic Press.

What do you have to do in your project to make yourself into a wise experimenter?

Imagine that you have written a new booklet which you believe will help patients to recover more quickly from a particular type of intervention, for example, surgery.

- How would you design an experiment to test the effectiveness of your booklet?
- What ethical problems might you have to consider?
- What factors might make it difficult to be sure about the validity of your experiment

Another word for 'paradigm' is 'pattern'. Think about the different patterns of research outlined on these pages.

How might these patterns influence your enquiry?

Do you feel more drawn to one pattern than another for your project?

treatment that they express on discharge.

One way of conducting an experiment is to test the subject before and after the intervention. If everything else remains the same, the implication is that any changes are caused by the intervention itself. The problem with this is that people will react to any kind of intervention, regardless of its actual value. So, a patient who is given a placebo drug may report an improvement in symptoms.

Another way to conduct an experiment is to divide a group of subjects into randomised groups. One group is exposed to the intervention. Other groups are exposed to no intervention at all, or to a different intervention. (In drug trials, a placebo may be given to one group.) In a true experiment, it is essential that the researcher is unaware of the group to which an individual subject has been assigned, because this knowledge could introduce other variables. This is known as a 'double blind' trial.

Surveys

In a survey, the researcher observes the effects of variables in a situation and does not try to manipulate them. For example, a survey might look at the age of people using a hospital canteen and compare this variable with the fat content of the food selected. Surveys raise fewer ethical dilemmas than experiments. Since they simply observe reality, rather than try to change it, researchers do not have to consider whether a particular intervention, or the lack of it, could damage their subjects. But they have less control of the variables they can observe, because they are not introducing them.

A survey, like an experiment, is based on a hypothesis. The design of a survey depends on the variables being investigated. It is quite possible to design a survey to test several hypotheses simultaneously. For example, researchers might want to investigate whether the fat content of food chosen in a canteen was related to the age, sex, or educational background of the subjects. Even so, the data gathered depends on the researcher's understanding of the situation before the survey begins. Suppose that there was actually a strong relationship between the nature of the physical work done by the subjects and the fat content of their meals. If the researcher had not thought of this before designing the questions, the information would probably not emerge from the survey.

An excellent introduction to the research process is:

Robson, C. (1993) *Real World Research*. Oxford: Blackwell.

Another key text, which concentrates on quantitative methods, is:

Polit, D. F. and Hungler, B. P. (1993) *Essentials of Nursing Research*. (3rd edition). Philadelphia: J.B. Lippincott Company.

There is a brief and very accessible introduction to experiments in the following article:

Sleep, J. (1990) An introduction to the experimental method. *Nursing Standard* 4(41): 34-36.

Some people, if they realise that a researcher is checking the fat content of the food they select for lunch at the canteen, might alter their choice of food.

- How could a researcher avoid any distortion of this kind?
- How much do you think that subjects should be told about the purpose of a survey?

The following article discusses whether experiments should continue to have a role in nursing research:

Wilson-Barnett, J. (1991) The experiment: Is it worthwhile? *International Journal of Nursing Studies* 28(1): 77-87.

A good practical introduction to qualitative research is:

Field, P. A. and Morse, J. M. (1995) *Nursing Research: The application of qualitative approaches*. London: Chapman and Hall.

Research paradigms — 2

Ethnography

Ethnography is often used in healthcare research. It is concerned with the role individuals play in society. A society can be as narrow as the home, or as broad as a village, workplace or any other social situation.

Ethnography evolved from anthropology and relies on the researchers immersing themselves in the social setting (known as the 'field') to develop an understanding of the cultural issues. Ethnographers try to understand the meanings that members of society attach to aspects of their daily life and how they develop an understanding of their world.

Information is collected and converted into data using a variety of methods. The most usual is to participate in the everyday activities of the social group, making careful records of observations and interrogating informants for explanation of the observed culture. Observations may trigger further investigations and the researcher may make use of documents such as hospital records, newspapers, case studies, life histories and professional journals.

The information collected in an ethnographic study is analysed by a process of coding. Researchers may be aware of some types of code before starting the analysis. Others will emerge as they look at the data in detail.

Ethnology is concerned with developing theories of culture and society. It is used to compare and contrast cultures. Ethnoscience (sometimes known as ethnolinguisitcs) is an attempt to introduce an objective approach to data generation through quantification or by applying procedures concerned with the structural analysis of language.

Grounded theory, originated by Glaser and Strauss (1967), is a way of analysing data used in ethnography. It involves checking the analysis of data by returning to the field. The researcher collects information in the field, analyses it for codes, themes and categories, writes descriptions of the categories and returns to the field to ask informants about the categories, which can then be verified or discarded. Grounded theory uses both inductive and deductive reasoning. A theory is obtained by analysing the data (inductive) and the theory is then tested out in the field (deductive).

'An ethnographer asks the question: 'In what ways do members of society actively construct their social world?'

'Translated into a nursing study, the researchers might ask: "What do nurses in a surgical unit see themselves as doing?" The researcher wants to find out what it is that one has to know in order to be accepted as a surgical nurse. What competencies must one have? What values must one hold to be accepted by other nurses in the group?'

Field, P.A. and Morse, J.M. (1985) *Nursing Research: The application of qualitative approaches.* London: Chapman and Hall.

Spradley, J.P. and McCurdy, D. (1972) *The Cultural Experience: Ethnography in complex society.* Chicago: Science Research Associates.

Here is a simple example of how grounded theory could work in practice:

A researcher talks to a group of nurses about the strategies they use with disruptive patients in an accident and emergency unit. She goes away and analyses her data and finds eight different strategies that seem to be in use. She then goes back to the nurses and asks them to comment on the categories she has identified. The nurses suggest that two of her categories should, in fact, be combined and that one of her categories can be sub-divided. The researcher amends her analysis accordingly.

If you would like to find more about grounded theory, key texts are:

Glaser, B. and Strauss, A. (1967) *The Discovery of Grounded Theory.* New York: Aldine de Gruyter.

Strauss, A. and Corbin T. (1990) *Basics of Qualitative Research: Grounded theory procedures and techniques.* Newbury Park, Ca.: Sage Publications Inc.

Phenomenology

The aim of phenomenology is to describe the essence of a life experience as lived by the individual. It answers questions such as: 'What does it feel like to be a patient in this situation?'

Data can be collected by interviewing informants or reading written accounts. Observation is not usually used. But supplementary data obtained from a variety of sources, such as literature or art, can be used to provide structure and shape to the participants' accounts.

Some phenomenologists prepare for the analysis by formulating their own definitions of the phenomenon and then looking through the data to support these definitions. Other researchers believe that it is essential to approach the analysis without pre-conceived definitions.

Emancipatory research

This type of research is based on the value of personal investigation and practical knowledge. The results may not be generalisable, but can empower individuals in their day-to-day living and working activities. There are various approaches:

Feminist research is concerned with issues of concern to women. A variety of methods is used, but in all of them efforts are made to change the traditional power relationship between researcher and researched.

Action research encourages individuals to take control of their own lives and create desirable change through systematic investigation into their own practice. It can also be concerned with evaluating and implementing change on an institutional level, in which case it may be conducted by a guest researcher working with the staff of the organisation. Another area of action research is concerned with investigating personal practice with the aim of developing new ways of operating effectively.
It is possible to give here only a very general introduction to the various research paradigms. Deepen your understanding by following up some of the suggestions for further reading.

The unit *Values and the Person: Ideas that influence health care* includes a description of phenomenology and other 'tools of mind' for thinking about health and health care.

It may help you to grasp the differences between the different paradigms if you think about them in terms of the area of study identified for your project. How could you use each of the paradigms to illuminate your topic?

'A feminist methodology of social science requires...that the mythology of "hygienic" research with its accompanying mystification of the researcher and the researched as objective instruments of data production be replaced by the recognition that personal involvement is more than a dangerous bias - it is the condition under which people come to know each other and to admit others to their lives.'

Oakley, A. (1981) Interviewing women. In: Roberts, H. *Doing Feminist Research*. London: Routledge and Kegan Paul.

An early example of phenomenological research is in:

Van Kaam, A.L. (1959) Phenomenological analysis: exemplified by a study of the experience of feeling really understood. *Journal of Individual Psychology* 15: (Part 1, May), 66-72.

A useful book on ethnography is:

Lincoln, Y. and Denzin, N. (1994) *The Handbook of Qualitative Research*. Newbury Park, Ca.: Sage Publications Inc.

You can find out more about feminist research in:

Webb, C. (1993) Feminist research: Definitions, methodology, methods and evaluation. *Journal of Advanced Nursing* 18: 416-423.

Roberts, H. (1981) *Doing Feminist Research*. London: Routledge and Kegan Paul.

You can find more about action research in nursing in:

Titchen, A. and Binnie, A. (1993) *Changing Nursing Practice Through Action Research*. Oxford: National Institute for Nursing.

A text which discusses action research in education is:

Elliot, J. (1991) *Action Research for Educational Change*. Milton Keynes: Open University Press.

Ways of knowing

The research paradigms described on the previous pages provide very different kinds of knowledge. In various ways, they all contribute to the development of professional understanding.

The four patterns of knowing described by Carper (1978) were introduced on page 24 in the context of structured reflection. It is useful to look at them in more detail now. While her model is used predominately in nursing, it can usefully be applied to all healthcare professions.

Empirical

This is the science of practice, concerned with developing theoretical explanations from verifiable facts. It includes:

- Physiological knowledge which informs practice, such as theories about how pressure sores develop or how babies develop immunity if they are breastfed
- Conceptual models, such as the representation of health as something more than the absence of disease.

Aesthetic

This is the art of practice and involves perception and empathy and an appreciation of the complexity of human behaviour. Aesthetics is difficult to define, but it is something that both patients and other health professionals can recognise when it is present. A professional who is aesthetically skilled will be able to pick up subtle cues and identify what is significant in a patient's behaviour, and act appropriately.

Personal

This refers to the nature of the interpersonal process between the professional and the patient. It goes beyond the empathy and perception involved in aesthetics to an awareness and acceptance of the uniqueness of the other individual. Carper says that personal knowledge is the most problematic pattern of knowing to master and to teach, but it is 'perhaps the pattern most essential to understanding the meaning of health in terms of individual well-being.' Personal knowing involves an understanding of oneself and the ability to respond intuitively to another person.

Ethical

The fourth way of knowing is concerned with having an appreciation of the moral component of healthcare practice. Codes of conduct and policy statements can provide some guidance, but ethical decisions also have to be made in

'. . . it is possible that the intuitive nurse is one who has resolved the difference between the academic and technical side of [the] profession and the practical and caring side. . . . Intuitive nurses are often more confident in their practice, as well as in their knowledge.'

Chapman, H. (1996) Why do nurses not make use of a solid research base? *Nursing Times*, 92 (3): 38-39.

'You know all the words and you learned the tune, but you never quite sang the song...'

(words from *The Hedgehog Song* by the Incredible String Band)

- Do you know any nurses to whom you could apply these lines?
- What is missing from their 'art' of nursing?

There is a section on aesthetics in the unit entitled *Values and the Person: Ideas that influence health care.*

Look at one of the models of structured reflection introduced on pages 22-25 and use it to describe an incident related to your enquiry topic.

- How did this incident change your ways of knowing?
- Would any of the research paradigms introduced in this Section help you increase your knowledge further?
- How would they help?

Individual practitioners should 'become more aware of... the knowledge which is gained through practice in interactions with others and in responding to the demands of situations in which it is not possible to draw on others' experience...[This] knowledge can be revealed through reflection. In reflection one looks at incidents critically, "replays" them in the imagination and tries to draw out what was learned and what was concluded in order to modify practice in the light of experience.'

Richardson, B. (1993) Practice, research and education – what is the link? *Physiotherapy* 79(5): 317-22.

ambiguous and uncertain situations, where you may not even be sure of the possible consequences of your actions.

Carper gives an example of the importance which is often attached to the goal of independence in patients. But, she asks, what value do you place on independence if a patient needs to come to accept a necessary degree of social or physical dependence?

Healthcare professionals need to understand the variety of philosophical standpoints and ethical frameworks which have been devised to help with moral decisions — and have the sensitivity and skill to apply them in specific situations.

Each of Carper's four patterns of knowing suggests a different kind of enquiry. For example, a researcher who is interested in investigating the treatment of myocardial infarctions might:
- Conduct a survey of the long-term effects of different forms of after-care (empirical)
- Conduct an ethnographic study of coping mechanisms used by partners (aesthetic)
- Conduct a piece of action research to improve the way stress control classes are run (personal)
- Conduct a phenomenological study of nurses' accounts of resuscitation (ethical).

These are just some of the possibilities. Other different ways of knowing include:
- Adversarial – as in the legal system
- Logical – as in mathematics and philosophy
- Judgemental – as in competitions and contests
- Demographic – as in economics
- Religious – as in all belief systems or faiths.

The decision about which research paradigm to use is based on the kind of knowledge researchers are looking for. For example:
- A survey or an experiment allows them to test out a hypothesis against observable data
- An ethnographic study may yield valuable insights into the beliefs of patients or other health professionals which will enable them to understand more about the art of practice and allow them to improve their own practice.

Some people find themselves more attracted to one paradigm than another. This may be because the paradigm reflects their own values and view of the world - or because they are used to the data collection methods involved.

'Nursing thus depends on the scientific knowledge of human behaviour in health and in illness, the aesthetic perception of significant human experiences, a personal understanding of the unique individuality of the self and the capacity to make choices within concrete situations involving particular moral judgements.'

Carper, B. (1978) Fundamental patterns of knowing in nursing. *Advances in Nursing Science* 1: 13-23.

Some possible routes from patterns of knowing to choice of enquiry methods

	Paradigm	*Methods*
Empirical	Positivism	Experiment or survey
Aesthetic	Ethnography Phenomenology	Observation and interview In-depth interview
Ethical	Phenomenology	Literature review
Personal	Emancipatory	Action research

Here is how one nurse rated herself on a scale of 0 to 5 on Carper's four patterns of knowing:

Empirical	*****	Personal	***
Aesthetic	****	Ethical	**

'I know the "mechanics" of the job inside out and can apply my knowledge pretty well with individual patients. Generally, my relationships with patients are good, although I find the personal distress of some patients hard to bear and tend to withdraw. The area where I feel least certain is in making choices about how much information I should disclose to a patient about their condition.'

- How would you rate yourself?
- What are the implications for your choice of research topic and method?

The issue of validity

A piece of research or enquiry is useful to other people only if they can be confident that it gives an accurate picture of reality. This is what is meant by the 'validity' of research.

Quantitative and qualitative research look at the world in different ways. Quantitative research tries to reduce a situation to a series of variables that can be measured and to establish cause and effect between different variables. Qualitative research tries to describe how a situation is perceived by the people involved in it. Not surprisingly, the concept of validity has different implications in these two branches of research.

Two kinds of validity have to be considered in quantitative research. Internal validity is the extent to which the study methods affect the results. For example, if a healthcare professional wanted to find out what her colleagues thought about a new managerial system, she wouldn't just ask friends for their views. She would question a representative sample of nurses using a carefully thought out set of questions designed to avoid bias.

External validity is concerned with how generalisable results and conclusions are to other situations. This is very important in quantitative research, where the aim is to look for universal laws. External validity can be affected by anything that makes the sample unique. If quantitative research is done in a real setting, such as a workplace, it can be difficult to make sure that other factors are not interfering with results. The reliability of methods of measurement can also affect validity.

When it comes to interpreting the results of a quantitative study, researchers need an understanding of statistics so they can establish the degree to which results may or may not be due to chance. It tends to be assumed that results with only a less than 20:1 probability of being due to chance are seen as significant (worthy of special note).

The validity of qualitative research

Subjectivity is unavoidable in qualitative research. This has led some people to dismiss the value of ethnographic and phenomenological studies. But in healthcare enquiry, subjectivity can be a strength not a weakness. Field and Morse (1985) describe two kinds of subjectivity that occur in qualitative research. First, the researcher cannot help affecting the quality of information that is

A study carried out by Duffy (1985), quoted earlier research by Campbell and Stanley (1963) who identified eight classes of extraneous variables which can be used to test the internal validity of an experiment:

1 *History:* other effects occurring during the study.
2 *Maturation:* changes within the respondents.
3 *Testing:* effects of taking one test on the second.
4 *Instrumentation:* changes in the instrument.
5 *Statistical regression:* sample selection on the basis of extreme scores.
6 *Selection biases:* effects of personal bias in sample selection.
7 *Experimental mortality:* loss of sample members.
8 *Interaction of extraneous variables:* selection-maturation.

They also identified four factors which can affect external validity in an experiment:

1. Reactive or interactive effects of testing in which pre-testing may sensitise the sample to the experimental variable.
2. Interaction effects of selection biases and the experimental variable.
3. Reactive effects of experimental arrangements which may alter the effects of the experimental variable in the non-experimental setting.
4. Multiple treatment interference since the effects of prior treatment cannot be eliminated.

Duffy, M.E. (1985) Designing nursing research: the qualitative-quantitative debate. *Journal of Advanced Nursing* 10: 225-232.

Campbell, D.T. and Stanley, J.C. (1963) *Experimental and Quasi-Experimental Design for Research.* Chicago: Rand McNally.

gathered in in-depth interviews and observation. If an interviewer does not manage to establish a good relationship with his or her subjects, they may not reveal important information. Second, 'the purpose of qualitative research is not to determine objectively what actually happened (as in a court of law) but rather to report objectively the perceptions of each of the actors in the setting.'

If you are using participant observation or interviewing, you need to consider:
- Do you have preconceptions which are distorting what you are seeing?
- Have you got adequate access to the people or events you are studying?
- Are you over-identifying with the subjects of your study?
- How much do you know about the topic?
- How much do the subjects know about the area you are studying and are they typical members of their group?
- How well do you relate to your subjects?
- Are your subjects behaving naturally?

Lincoln and Guba (1985) argue that the criteria of validity and reliability cannot be applied to qualitative research. Instead, they suggest that the researcher should be concerned with four other criteria: credibility, transferability, dependability and confirmability.

Credibility can be increased by prolonged engagement, persistent observation, triangulation, peer debriefing, negative case analysis, referential adequacy (checking preliminary findings and interpretations against raw data) and member checking (checking findings and interpretations with your research subjects).

Transferability, for qualitative researchers, does not mean that their findings can be transferred to other settings. It means that the researcher should provide sufficient data, or 'thick description' so that others can decide whether any transfer is possible.

Dependability is the qualitative equivalent of reliability. Dependability and confirmability can both be established by an audit trail — a method of checking the processes and products of a study.

'Measure quantitatively that which should be quantified; measure qualitatively that which should not be quantified.'

Senge, P. ed. (1994) *The Fifth Discipline Fieldbook.* London: Nicholas Brearley Publishing.

Use some of the reflective techniques described in Section 1 to think about the preconceptions you bring to your research. Could this affect the way you collect and analyse the data, and how you interpret the results?

You can find out more about validity and reliability in:

Sandelowski, M. (1986) The problem of rigour in qualitative research. *Advances in Nursing Science* 8(3): 27-37.

Lincoln, Y.S. and Guba, E.G. (1985) *Naturalistic Inquiry.* Newbury Park, Ca.: Sage Publications Inc. (This book also contains Edward S. Halpern's description of how to set up an audit trail.)

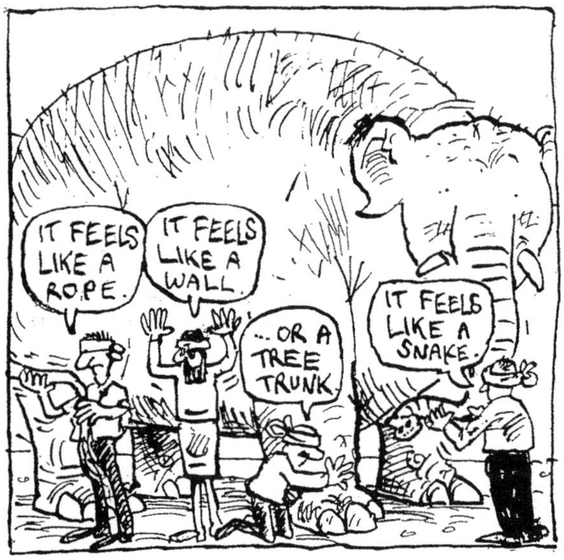
IT FEELS LIKE A ROPE.
IT FEELS LIKE A WALL.
...OR A TREE TRUNK
IT FEELS LIKE A SNAKE.

TIM SAUNDERS

On reflection...

The language of research

When you start to read about the theory of research, you may come across some unfamiliar terminology. Many people find this technical vocabulary quite off-putting.

Some words, such as 'phenomenology' and 'ethnography', are usually used only in the context of academic work. You will also meet words which are used in everyday life, but have a specialised meaning. For example, 'population' is used by statisticians to mean a set of objects or individuals with some characteristic in common.

One source of confusion is that some words are used slightly differently by various authors. For example, a study that you would consider to be an example of phenomenology might be described as ethnographic research. This kind of disagreement is inevitable among people who are exploring the frontiers of their subject. Be aware of differences between definitions and use them to build up your own understanding.

On the opposite page you will find explanations of some of the technical terms you may encounter in your reading about research techniques.

If you come across other terms note them down on this page, with a brief description.

When you were a young child first learning to speak, you would hear a word such as 'tractor' and use it when you next saw something that fitted your idea of what a tractor was. If you were right, an adult would reinforce your use of the word by congratulating you. If you used the word inappropriately, an adult would notice and correct your mistake.

Now that you are an adult, what strategies do you use to learn new vocabulary?

Many standard textbooks on research contain glossaries. Use them to look up individual words, and also browse through them occasionally. You may be surprised at the definitions of some terms that you thought you understood.

It can be very helpful to build up your own personal glossary as you do your research. You might like to do this in your reflective journal.

Writing things down is a good way to extend and expand language.

'Language inherently involves sharing a code with other people.'

Pinker, S. (1994) *The Language Instinct*. London: Penguin.

Terms commonly used in research

Basic research: concerned with generating new knowledge

Concept: a mental image or generalisation of an object, property or event that is derived from individual perceptual experience. Concepts can be concrete (specific to time or place) or abstract (independent of time and place)

Cross-sectional study: a study that examines subjects at one point in time

Data: pieces of information or facts that are collected in a research study

Deduction: a form of reasoning that moves from the general to the specific.

Determinism: causal explanation, the belief that events have causes and are determined by circumstances and are thus understandable if the law that governs their behaviour can be found

Emancipatory: the use of the interpretative process, with the belief that the process will empower the people who are subjects of the research

Epistemology: theory of knowledge

Experimental study: a study in which the researcher manipulates or controls the independent variable (cause) and observes the dependent variable (effect)

Grand theory: a theory that is broad in scope and complexity, usually needing further specification before it can be tested

Hypothesis: a statement that predicts the relationship between two or more variables

Independent variable: the 'cause'; the variable that is thought to influence the dependent variable

Induction: a form of reasoning that moves from the specific to the general

Interpretative research: research that aims to discover the meanings held by an individual and thus what is particular and unique, rather than general

Knowledge: an awareness or perception of reality acquired through learning or investigation

Laboratory study: the study of subjects in a special environment that has been created by the researchers

Metaphysics: first principles of nature/thought; the science of investigating the ultimate reality

Model: an idea explained through symbolic and physical visualisation or through more abstract means, such as language or mathematics

Population: a group of individual people or objects who share certain characteristics

Post-structuralist: a perspective in which it is assumed that knowledge equals power and thus the knowledge must be located with the subject(s) of the research rather than the investigator

Qualitative study: concerned with in-depth descriptions of people or events, collected through such methods as unstructured interviews and participant observation

Quantitative research: concerned with numbers and other data that can be converted into numbers

Retrospective study: the dependent variable is identified in the present (eg a disease condition) and an attempt is made to determine the independent variable

Sample: a sub-group of the population, chosen to represent the population and used to make generalisations about the population under study

Science: the systematic and objective study of phenomena, based traditionally on observation, experiment and measurement

Survey: a type of non-experimental research that focuses on obtaining information regarding the status quo of some situation, often through direct questioning or a sample of respondents

Target population: the group of people or objects to which the researcher wishes to generalise the findings of a study

Theory: a set of concepts, definitions and propositions that project a systematic view of phenomena by demonstrating specific

Conclusion

This Section introduced the main approaches used to research or enquire into healthcare practice today. It showed how research resembles, and also differs from, the kinds of enquiry you make in your ordinary life and as part of your everyday professional role.

Research can be divided into qualitative and quantitative studies. Within these two branches, a range of different paradigms exists, including experiments, surveys, ethnography, phenomenology and emancipatory research (which includes action and feminist research).

You should now have an understanding of how different approaches can be used to address various types of question. Section 4 shows how to make a decision appropriate to the type of enquiry you are going to undertake.

Use your learning journal or reflective diary to record your thoughts about the different forms of research and how each might be relevant to your own topic of enquiry.

References

Carlson, M. and Clark, F. (1991) The search for useful methodologies in occupational science. *American Journal of Occupational Therapy* 45(3): 235-41.

Carper, B. (1978) Fundamental patterns of knowing in nursing. *Advances in Nursing Science* 1: 13-23.

Chapman, H. (1996) Why do nurses not make use of a solid research base? *Nursing Times*, 92(3): 38-39.

Christiansen, C. (1991) Research: looking back and ahead after four decades of progress. *American Journal of Occupational Therapy* 45(5): 391-393.

DHSS (1972(a)) *Report of the Committee on Nursing.* (Briggs Report). London: HMSO.

DHSS (1972(b)) *A Framework for Government Research and Development.* (White Paper). London: HMSO.

DoH (1993[a]). *Report of the Taskforce on a Strategy for Research in Nursing, Midwifery and Health Visiting.* London: HMSO.

DoH (1993[b]). *Research for Health.* London: DoH.

DoH (1991). *The Health of the Nation. A consultative document for health in England.* London: HMSO, Cmnd 1523.

Field, P.A. and Morse, J.M. (1985) *Nursing Research: The application of qualitative approaches.* London: Chapman and Hall.

Glaser, B. and Strauss, A. (1967) *The Discovery of Grounded Theory.* New York: Aldine de Gruyter.

Hopps, L. C. (1994) The development of research in nursing in the United Kingdom. *Journal of Clinical Nursing* 3(4): 199-204.

Inman, U. (1975) *Towards a Theory of Nursing Care.* London: Royal College of Nursing.

Lincoln Y.S. and Guba E.G. (1985) *Naturalistic Inquiry.* Newbury Park, Ca.: Sage Publications Inc.

Mosey, A.C. (1971) Occupational therapy - a historical perspective. *American Journal of Occupational Therapy* 25: 234-236.

NHS Research and Development Task Force. *Supporting Research and Development in the NHS* (the Culyer Report). London: HMSO, 1994.

Polit, D.F. and Hungler, B.P. (1993) *Essentials of Nursing Research* (3rd edition). Philadelphia: J.B. Lippincott Company.

Richardson, B. (1993) Practice, research and education - what is the link? *Physiotherapy* 79(5): 317-22.

Royal Commission on the National Health Service (1979). (Chairman Sir Alec Merrison.) London: HMSO. Cmnd 7615.

Introduction

Very few pieces of research or enquiry break completely new ground. Most studies relate in different ways to preceding research - and researchers benefit from the process of reading around and into the subject. Your enquiry-based project should be set in the context of what is already known about the topic. Your assessors will look for evidence that you are familiar with the relevant literature.

Academic books and research journals are not the only sources of information. Current policies and procedures relevant to your area of interest may be just as important, especially if you are enquiring into aspects of management or structural change.

This Section explains how to conduct a literature search and describes some techniques you can use when reading books and journals and when taking notes. There are also guidelines for reading research reports and suggestions for the kinds of questions you should be asking when looking at statistical information.

'We return to the importance of the questioning attitude of mind. Ask yourself questions such as the following:

- Why did that happen?
- What is the connection between this and that?
- How is that known?
- What is the evidence for this assertion?
- What follows?
- How is it that so and so is the case when something else is the case; is there no consistency?
- What other examples are there of this sort of thing happening; does it illustrate any general rule?
- What is the history of this?

Let your questions come. Try to get them clear, then follow their lead as far as ever they will go. And then, ask yourself another question.'

Mace, C. A. (1962) *The Psychology of Study*. London: Pelican.

Sources of information

When you have clarified a topic for enquiry and agreed its scope with your tutor/counsellor, the next stage is to find out about existing knowledge on the subject. This will allow you to learn from earlier research and put your own findings in context.

Your assessor will want to see that you have performed a thorough review of the academic literature relevant to your area of study. Many students think that this part of their research is a necessary formality with no real practical purpose. But it has important benefits.

The following reasons for carrying out a literature review were listed by Leedy (1989). Literature reviews can:

- Reveal investigations similar to your own, and show you how the researcher handled these situations
- Suggest a method or a technique for dealing with a problematic situation which may help you solve similar difficulties
- Reveal sources of data that you may not have known existed
- Introduce you to significant research
- Help you to see your own study in perspective and in relation to earlier investigations of the same problem
- Provide new ideas and approaches which may not have occurred to you
- Help you to evaluate your own research efforts by comparing them with related efforts done by others.

More information on how to conduct and record a literature review is given in the rest of this Section.

After completing your project you may find that the research literature surrounding your area of work has become more accessible and interesting. From time to time, use some of the techniques described in the following pages to investigate other issues. Your personal profile is a good place to keep track of your investigations.

As well as a formal literature review, you could also usefully explore other sources of information, such as the ones listed here:

- Are there any healthcare professionals who are working in the same research area as you? They may not have published their findings in academic journals, but they might be running

Sometimes people remember a particular book or article they have read which has given them significant new insights into their work.

If you wanted to recommend a book or article to your colleagues:

- What would it be?
- Why would you choose it?

List the journals and other publications relevant to your enquiry topic.

- What benefits will you expect to get from reading them?
- How will you make judgements about articles - will you have a subjective response, or will you look for ways of taking an objective viewpoint?

Here is a list of headings drawn up by one student to help her make notes on literature she reads:

- Statement of problem
- Literature referred to
- Theoretical concepts introduced
- Assumptions
- Type of study
- Aims of the study
- Population and sample
- Methodology
- Ethical considerations
- Analysis and results
- Conclusions and recommendations.

seminars for interested professionals and could be very happy to talk to you. Look out for reports in the healthcare press and ask your colleagues. Your tutor/counsellor may also be aware of people you could contact

- Talk to colleagues in different disciplines. They may know about work in their own field that is relevant to your study
- Talk to friends and, if appropriate, patients or clients. They may have useful observations and insights for you
- It may be that the issue you are interested in has been covered in some way in the national media. Quality newspapers, television and radio can sometimes give useful leads
- There may be guidelines or policy statements issued by the NHS or your local health authority that relate to your study
- Are there any organisations, such as charities or associations, which work in the same field as your study? They may be engaged in research, employ people who are well briefed about current developments or have library facilities you could use
- Think about experiences you have had yourself which may be relevant to your area of study. Your reflective journal may be a source of ideas.

The information you get from these sources may be anecdotal or incomplete. But it could give you new perspectives and suggest areas for more formal enquiry.

You may find yourself able to link up with a network of healthcare professionals who are interested in your area of study. It is quite possible that they will be interested in the contribution your project could make to their own understanding.

Here are the results of an initial exercise which one student undertook to think of possible sources of information for her project about the care of HIV/AIDS patients in the community.

- Local authority guidelines
- Discharge procedures
- Social services department
- Terrence Higgins Trust
- Needle Exchange - researcher who visited them last year could provide leads?
- My friend Robert (buddy system)
- Case reported in press about European nationals not being allowed to stay.

Think of your existing knowledge of your chosen topic as an incomplete jigsaw.

- What is missing from the picture?
- Where do you need to extend your knowledge?
- What seems to fit together?

Brainstorm sources of information about your own topic. Your tutor/counsellor is likely to be a good source of information if you get stuck. And don't ignore serendipity — making fortunate discoveries by accident.

Starting a literature review

The standard method of searching the literature has five stages.

1. Identify as many texts as possible which may be relevant to your subject, by consulting databases, indices and abstracts.
2. When you have identified a relevant text, list the details. This was traditionally done on a card index system, although there are many advantages of using a computer database (see page opposite).
3. Obtain the texts, read them and make notes.
4. Identify the important references quoted in these texts and add them to your list.
5. Select the central material and, in your literature review, describe and criticise the ideas it contains.

The literature you are investigating is not a series of unrelated items. If an article or book is important to the subject, by definition it will have influenced the thinking of other people: it is very rare to find a text that is completely original. Most writers build their work on foundations laid by others. Like you, they assess existing ideas and theories and add their own developments. Since it is accepted practice for writers to quote their sources, as this book does, you will find that any significant text will lead you on to others. This principle is exploited in the alternative method of researching the literature described on pages 64 and 65.

How to find the literature

Your library may subscribe to an indexing service which lists books and articles in relevant fields. New editions are published monthly, bi-monthly or quarterly. Useful indexes are:

- Cumulative Index of Nursing and Allied Health Literature (CINAHL)
- Index Medicus
- International Nursing Index (INI)
- Chartered Society of Physiotherapists.

Abstracting services provide summaries of articles. They do not usually cover quite as many titles as in an index and are not updated so regularly. But they are a very useful way of knowing whether an article is relevant to your needs before you go to the trouble of finding a copy.

A useful abstracting service is:

- Health Service Abstracts, published by the Department of Health.

Key texts are suggested in this book and in other books in the degree programme. These texts have been selected to give useful entry points into the literature and are well worth following up.

An invaluable book which contains references, with brief descriptions, on almost every aspect of the research process, is:

Clamp, C. (1994) *Resources for Nursing Research: An annotated bibliography*. London: Library Association Publishing.

'The good student has a reverence for books. The better student is more critical of books. He asks for their credentials.'

Mace, C. A. (1969) *The Psychology of Study*. London: Pelican.

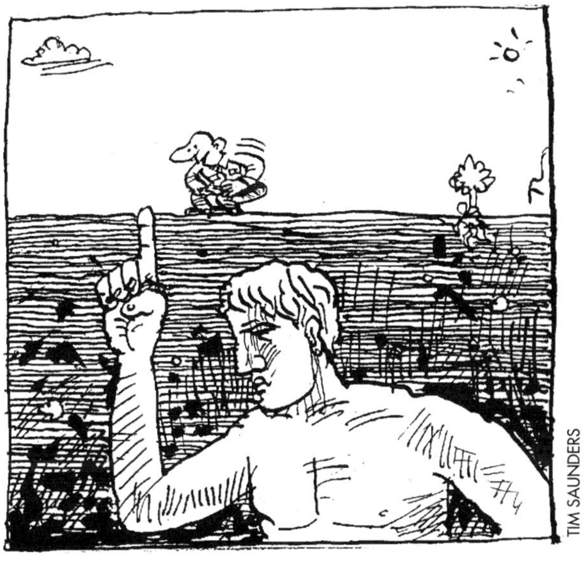
TIM SAUNDERS

A literature search is a bit like archaeology. Once you start to dig, you may find yourself unearthing a whole connected structure

Computer technology has revolutionised the process of searching the literature. Many indices and abstracts are now available on CD-ROM, which makes them quicker to search. You can usually search by title, author or key words.

There are also several online databases which you can access. The Royal College of Nursing (RCN) is making the CINAHL index available online. The English National Board (ENB) also has an online healthcare database.

In order to get access to an online service, you need a computer with a modem. Sometimes you will also need special software. Many online services are free, but others charge per search or per item.

How to get hold of the literature
It makes sense to start with the most convenient sources - probably a college or hospital library. There may be more comprehensive libraries in other local centres that you can arrange to use. Libraries can borrow books and journals from other collections. This can take some time, so don't leave your literature search until the last minute.

If you know there is a journal article which is absolutely central to your work but which your library does not have, you can usually arrange to have a copy faxed to you by one of the online services. Some of these services also allow you to download the text of articles directly onto your computer. It can be quite expensive and is not a substitute for normal library services. But in particular situations, you may feel the cost is worth it.

The amount of material available online is growing all the time. A good way to find out what is available is to make contact on the Internet with other researchers in your field.

With access to a suitably equipped computer, you can make informal links with other researchers through the Internet. If you can find a forum where other professionals congregate, it can be an extra source of support and information. Here is part of a conversation between healthcare professionals in Canada and the UK engaged in research on a similar issue.

Subj: Nursing Research Section: Nursing
To: Richard

Yes, I had that problem too. Held me up for weeks. Have you come across the work at Bristol? They were looking at staff perceptions. It might be relevant.

Sarah

Subj: Nursing Research Section: Nursing
To: Sarah

Could you give me a reference for that Bristol study? Also anything else you found useful. I've reached a dead end here and would really appreciate some leads.

Richard

Subj: Nursing Research Section: Nursing
To: Richard

Sure, I'd be glad to help. I have a copy of my references for the paper I've just submitted. I'll send the whole list.

Sarah

Find out about the sources of information available to you in local libraries.

- To which journals do they subscribe?
- What indices and abstracts do they have?
- How often are they updated?
- What arrangements do they make for inter-library loans?
- How long does it take?

Talk to your librarian and find out if there are any other facilities or training sessions offered to students.

An alternative approach

The purpose of a literature review is to find out what research has been done in and around your topic. You need to show how ideas have developed over time, how one writer built on the work of another and how your own findings fit in with what is already known.

You can obtain the information you need by following the standard method described on the previous two pages. But this process does have its disadvantages.

Computer databases make the initial search much easier and quicker than it used to be, but the standard method is still very time consuming. You will also probably have to read through a lot of irrelevant material before isolating the central articles and texts. Another difficulty is that before you have a developed a 'feel' for what is important, you may miss or underestimate important ideas. Also, you may not read your sources in the most helpful order.

These problems with the standard method were described by O'Connor (1992) who offered another method, the Network theory, based on work by Ryan et al. (1991) which was in turn developed from a theory by Hesse (1980).

Network theory

O'Connor (1992) suggests that network theory can be used to identify the development of key ideas through the literature. This method allows you to form an overall picture of what has been written about your subject which you can then investigate more closely.

It is based upon the principle described by Ryan et al. (1991), that most articles have one, two and sometimes three core themes that can be traced back to earlier articles. The first step in unravelling the network is to make a chart showing how a recent selection of articles drew upon earlier writings (described in detail on the opposite page).

Once you have completed a chart, you can simplify it. As O'Connor explains, if article A refers to articles B and C, and article B also refers to C, you can disregard the connection between A and C, as your chart already shows a connection between A and C (through B).

By the end, your chart will probably show a few texts which seem central to the development of the literature. If a large number of writers quote a particular reference, shown by a large number

These two comments are from students who completed their literature review using the standard method:

'A search of the database threw up more than 200 articles - far more than I had time to read, and I didn't know which of them were the most important.'

'Because I didn't know what the key concepts were in the area, I didn't know what I was looking for and so missed some central texts.'

What problems have you experienced when searching for information on a new subject?

Online information managers sometimes use the idea of threads to help trace ideas and discussions through messages posted in a forum. If you are searching databases, you may find that the system tracks your route through. Like the ball of thread that Ariadne gave Theseus to guide him out of the labryinth, a tracking system can help you retrace your route and find the connections that led you from one item to another.

of lines on your chart, it makes sense to assume that this is an important reference.

By looking at how one article built upon ideas in earlier articles, you can see the forward development of ideas that you will need to describe in your literature review.

Charting

- Identify a small number, perhaps two or three, of the leading journals in the specific subject area
- Obtain back issues for the previous year. If the specific subject is not well documented, the previous two years will be required
- Identify the articles in these journals that relate to the subject area
- Starting with the most recent article, isolate from the text the key ideas and from the reference section the key texts that are drawn upon. Now chart the first article and those upon which it draws, as follows:
- On a large piece of blank paper (A3 at least) draw a graph with time (usually in years) on the 'X' axis and the articles on the 'Y' axis. The location of the article on the 'Y' axis is arbitrary - give yourself enough space to add more references. Allow enough space on the 'X' axis to chart more than one article in each year - the 'X' axis divisions do not have to be equi-distant
- Join the source article by a straight line to key references, which are similarly charted
- By charting the articles in reverse order of publication a complex picture of the relationships between articles and ideas can be built up
- Articles that are frequently referred to can then be read, and by the same process their antecedents can be identified and charted
- The process continues until the roots of the subject matter have been identified, or the key references noted
- Early in the process there is a tendency for all the references to be charted, but after a short space of time, as the material becomes more familiar, key references and eventually only the central ideas come to be charted.

O'Connor, S.E. (1992) Network theory - a systematic method for literature review: *Nurse Education Today* 12: 44-50.

Look at these patterns.

- Which do you think represents a seminal article and which a review article?
- Which would you want to read first?

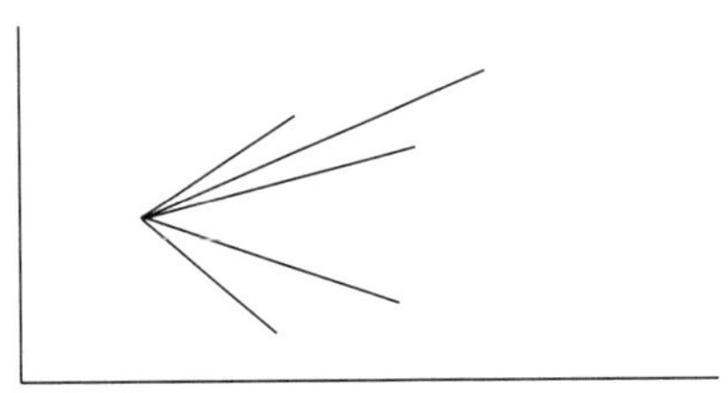

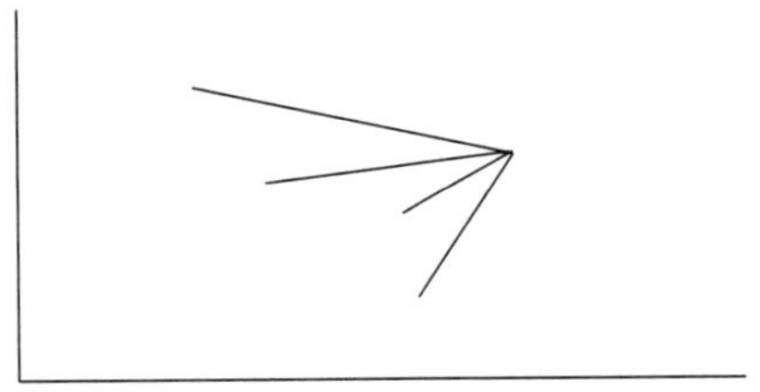

Which technique (standard or network theory) will you use when you do your literature review?

Reading techniques

When you first look at the reading ahead of you, and the complexity of some of the material involved, you might feel daunted by the amount there is to do. But you can make it a lot easier for yourself. In everyday life, we get into the habit of reading books from cover to cover, giving equal attention to every paragraph. This is not an appropriate technique to use when gathering information for your project.

You already possess other reading skills which you can use on the literature.

Scanning, skimming and careful reading

Scanning is what you do when you let your eye run down a column of print until you see a significant word. You scan a telephone directory to find the name you are looking for. Scanning is useful when you are checking to see whether something is worth reading in more detail.

Skimming involves looking quickly through a text to pick out the main ideas. If you get a letter telling you whether or not you have succeeded in getting an interview for a new job, you would probably skim it quickly to get the general meaning of what it said before reading it more slowly. Skimming is useful if you think that something is giving you information which you already know something about. You are just looking for the new bits.

Careful reading is just what it says. It means giving a text your full critical attention, thinking about what the writer is saying and the implications of this message.

It is very useful if you can switch between these three reading techniques. For example, you could scan an article until you found a word which indicated that the author was discussing a subject of interest to you. You could skim the relevant section until you found an idea which challenged you, and then slow down and read the section carefully.

Signposts

Most books and articles have built-in signposts which will help you locate useful information. Get used to scanning the contents pages and indexes of books before you start reading. Research articles usually begin with an abstract or brief summary of their contents. They usually end with conclusions which draw together the preceding discussion. You can also make use of the subheadings and any significant passages

When you next read a magazine, notice the techniques you use to find the parts you want to read in detail. Do you read differently when you are looking for information and when you are reading for pleasure?

Think about keeping a reading log to record:

- Your responses to things you read
- The ideas that are stimulated by them
- Questions that arise.

'He has only half learned the art of reading who has not added to it the even more refined accomplishments of skipping and skimming.'

Lord Balfour, quoted in: Cohen, J.M. and Cohen, M.J. (1971) *A Dictionary of Modern Quotations*. London: Penguin.

This is what one academic researcher does in order to keep up with current research:

'When I see a research article that looks interesting, I sit down and read the summary and the conclusions, then glance through the subheadings and read the relevant parts in more detail. All the time my mind is ticking away. I'm thinking "Yes, yes. I know that. I've read that research report you're quoting, too...But what have you got to say about X's theory?"

'If I come to something that's new to me, I may read it several times to make sure I really understand what the author is saying. Quite often I'll put the journal down and think for a minute or so. It often helps to put the argument into my own words, as though I was explaining it to someone else.'

The Unit *Influences in Health Care: Media perspectives* examines the way people read different sorts of material. It encourages readers to think about the way things are written and to question everything – including what is written in these units!

which are picked out in larger type. Once you have an overview of what the article is saying, you will be able to interpret the detail more quickly.

SQ3R

This is a reading technique which is often recommended to students. The initials stand for:

- *Survey* - start by using scanning and skimming to find out what the text has to say which is relevant to your needs
- *Question* - think of questions you would like the author to answer for you in the text (see page 69 for suggestions about the kinds of questions to ask)
- *Read* - read only as much of the text as you need for your questions to be answered
- *Recall* - stop reading and make notes on the main points you have read, using your own language, not the language of the author
- *Review* - later, go through your notes and check if you still understand them and whether they answer your original questions.

The purpose of the notes you take is to increase your attention while you are reading, not to reproduce large sections of the text.

The trick is to keep your own needs firmly in mind when you are reading, and not to be sidetracked by other issues.

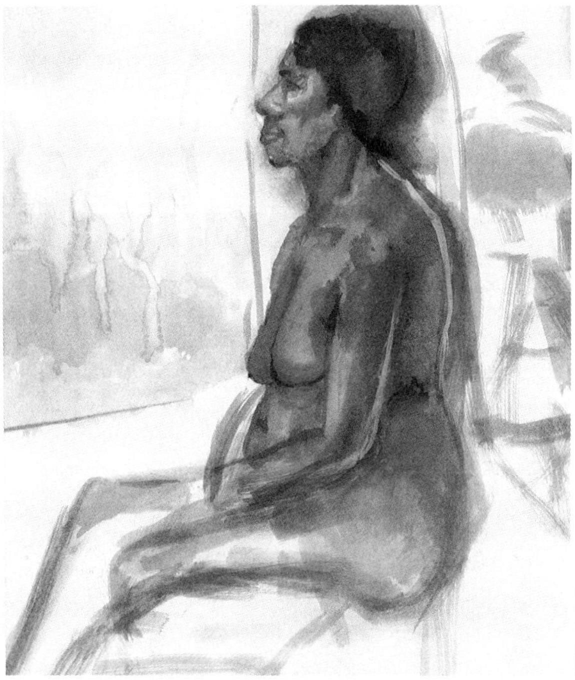

CATHY LAKE

'I constantly ask questions about what I am seeing' - one artist's approach to drawing

This is how an artist describes how she tackles a drawing. Can you see any parallels with the SQ3R technique?

'When I draw a model from life, I first get an overall impression of the shape of the figure and block it in very roughly on the paper. That gives me my bearings for the drawing. Then I look at particular areas in more detail.

'As I work, I constantly ask questions about what I am seeing. Is the arm in front of the leg or behind it? How exactly does that elbow bend? I try to work out the relationships between shapes while I am looking at the figure, so that I can reproduce them on paper. Then I check back, comparing the details of my drawing with the figure.'

Keep the topic and title of your project in the front of your mind as you read. It is a good idea to write it on a large piece of paper and stick it on the wall behind the desk where you work.

Reading should be an active process, in which you set the agenda, not a passive process in which you simply absorb information. This can be quite difficult because printed words carry a certain authority. We get used to accepting what we read - even though it may contradict our own experience. You will get much more out of your reading if you imagine yourself in a dialogue with the author.

Try out the SQ3R technique for yourself. Some people find it helpful to imagine they are reading the text on behalf of someone else. Pretend that a colleague has asked you if the text has anything important to say on a particular topic and summarise the main points of what you read so that you can report back.

Critical reading

Most people believe most of what they read, most of the time. Unless you have personal experience which directly contradicts what you are reading, you probably accept the author's version of reality. The respect that you give to the printed word probably dates back to early childhood and is a difficult habit to break. But, as a researcher, you have to develop a more critical attitude to what you read. This is particularly important if you are going to make changes to your practice based on your reading. A critical attitude should also make the actual process of reading much more stimulating and enjoyable.

As you read, challenge the writer with questions:

- Is there any possibility of bias here?
- Are you being selective with the facts?
- What is the main point you are making?
- Can you back up that statement?
- Does that argument really hold water?

Be aware of where the writer is coming from and also be conscious of any preconceptions and attitudes that you bring to the text. If you find a particular writer difficult, examine where the difficulty lies. It might be that the writing itself is hard. Or maybe you are finding the subject difficult to focus on for some reason. If so, you might want to try and find out the reason.

A critical attitude to reading does not mean that you set yourself up as an instant expert on the subject. The writers of most of the texts you read may have a great deal more experience and knowledge of the subject than you do. But that doesn't mean you have to accept everything they say. You may find faults in their logic or be aware of other factors they should have taken into account.

Reading research reports

In the panel on the opposite page is a list of questions to think about when reading a research report. If a report cannot stand up to this kind of scrutiny, it may be that its conclusions cannot be taken seriously.

'Just because it is written down does not mean it is research. Just because the author quotes Bloggs (1992) as "showing" something, does not mean that Bloggs did any original research.'

Griffiths, P. (1993) To believe or not to believe. *Nursing Times* 89(1): 39.

John Dewey, the philosopher and educationist wrote:

'A class of experts is inevitably so removed from common interests as to become a class with private knowledge, which in social matters is not knowledge at all.'

Quoted in Phillips, A. (1995) *Terrors and Experts*. London: Faber and Faber.

Chairman Mao is quoted as saying: 'The more books you read, the more stupid you become'.

Do you accept everything you read in this book? You shouldn't!

'I have a thing about sociological jargon. Whenever I see an 'ism' or a construct I want to shut off. It makes it difficult for me to read quite a lot of the material I know probably contains useful points.'

'It irritates me when male academics write about nursing when I know they got out of the real work of the profession as quickly as they could. Basically, I find it hard to take men seriously when they write about nursing.'

What preconceptions or prejudices do you bring to your reading of the literature?

A guideline for critiquing research reports

Research problem or question
- What is the research question?
- What is the researcher trying to find out?
- Is the problem/purpose clearly stated?

Rationale for the study
- What is the purpose of the study?
- Is it relevant to healthcare practice?
- Does the researcher make explicit the aims of the study?

Literature review
- Is there a comprehensive summary of related literature?
- Are positive and negative arguments presented?
- What is the time frame for the references?
- Is there evidence of wide reading?
- Are assumptions made?
- If so, are they justified and explained?
- Do hypotheses, relationships or questions emerge naturally from the literature review?
- Is there evidence of a theoretical framework?

Methodology
- Is the methodology explicit within the study?
- Is it placed within a quantitative or qualitative paradigm?
- Is it the appropriate methodology for the study?

Methods
- Subjects: How were they selected? Is the population identified and described? What was the response rate? Were refusals followed up? Did subjects give informed consent?
- How were the data collected? Who collected the data? Were assistants properly trained?
- What research tools are used? Are there reasons given for the choice of method? Is this explained in sufficient detail? Is there an example of the questionnaire/interview schedule?
- Is the issue of reliability and validity explored?
- Was there a pilot study? What, if any, were the changes?
- Is this a replication study? If so, is it a partial replication and what are the changes in this study from the original? Why were the changes made?

Results
- Did you have enough information to enable you to understand the data?
- Do you detect bias?
- Is the analysis appropriate to the study? Are statistical tests used?
- Are the results presented in a clear and unambiguous way?
- Do tables/graphs etc. summarise the results? Are they helpful?
- Are 'raw' figures always given if results are expressed in percentages?

Discussion/interpretation of results
- Are all the results discussed? Is the discussion reasonable and based on actual results?
- Are the aims of the study achieved?
- Were any inferences drawn from the study and are they justifiable?
- Was the interpretation linked to the original aims?
- Did the findings or results relate to previous research findings?
- Does the researcher discuss both expected and unexpected results?
- Were the results generalised to the population? Is this acceptable?
- Are the results biased because of interest of a financing body?
- Are suggestions made for implementing the results?
- Are limitations discussed?
- Are there suggestions made for further research? Are these appropriate? Are they realistic?

Implications
- Are there recommendations made for action?
- Are they discussed in terms of findings for healthcare practice, education and further research?
- Are they reasonable? Are they appropriate?
- What conclusions, if any, were drawn? Are they justified?

Recording a literature search

You probably won't have all the books and articles you want to read in your possession at one time. Many texts are in great demand and libraries issue them only for a limited period. You may also consult some reference sources that you are not allowed to take away from the library. So get into the habit of recording the information you need as you go along.

Record details of any book or article you have read or are thinking of reading, even though you may not include all the titles in your final review of the literature. Get into the habit of writing down a reference in full - it is irritating and time-consuming to look up the details later. As well as writing down the author and initials, title, date, publisher and place of publication of a work (and volume, issue and page numbers of a journal), write a brief comment which will help you bring the text to mind again. For example, if you have references for several articles on qualitative research techniques, it is useful to see at a glance which of them gives a comprehensive description of how to write field notes.

If you record your literature search on computer, you could use a database package. This will allow you to sort and retrieve titles more easily. You could also make full use of the database's facilities by devising a system of key words, allowing you to call up all the titles on your list which have something to say about a topic — for example, 'experimental techniques' or 'primary nursing'.

Taking notes

Most people take too many notes. It is tempting to try to write a simplified version of a chapter or article, but it doesn't help you much. Note-taking can become a substitute for understanding. You may find yourself writing down a lot of irrelevant information which you will never need to read again.

In the SQ3R technique, described on page 67, you read and understand the necessary parts of the text, put the book aside and then make notes. This means that taking notes does not distract attention from the text but is a way of fixing and recording your insights.

You may come across crucial sentences which you want to record for future quotation. In the SQ3R technique, these can be incorporated into your notes at the point when you review them.

One way of recording references

Author(s)	Title	Date	Publisher and place of publication (not necessary if a journal)	Comments
O'Connor, S. E.	Network theory - a systematic method for literature review. *Nurse Education Today*, 12, 44-50	1992		An interesting way of organising a literature search
Field, P.A. and Morse, J. M.	*Nursing Research: The application of qualitative approaches*	1985	London: Chapman & Hall	Essential reading for anyone engaged in qualitative research

The review stage is when you are in the best position to judge which are the central points made in the text. If you can, avoid the temptation to gather too much material for quoting. Two or three well chosen sentences from an article will probably be enough.

The traditional method of making notes is to write brief paragraphs on the different points you want to remember. It can be more effective if you use headings and subheadings to indicate the underlying structure. Arranging related points in a list can be an improvement on a long sentence.

You could abandon a linear structure altogether. Many people find it liberating to let the form of their notes mirror the form of their thinking and use spider diagrams or mind maps for their notes.

If you have bought a book or obtained a photocopy of an article, you may like to write your notes on the page itself (some ways of doing this are suggested below). If you are using a library book, or a book you don't want to mark, you could use small self-adhesive notes to make notes on the important pages.

The disadvantage of marking a text is that you don't go through the same process of distillation as you do when you write separate notes. It is very easy to mark every other sentence and, when you return to the book, find you are unable to identify the central points.

'Once you have got your book what should you do with it? The one thing you should not do is read it passively. If you have bought it, write in it! Annotate the margins, develop a system of notation, coloured underlining etc. which allows you to identify key passages, points you agree with, points you disagree with, errors of logic, empirical illustrations, bits you don't understand. Don't resort to the homogeneous yellow highlighter. In six months time you won't remember why you marked the passage.'

Advice to sociology students from Colin Mills, Department of Sociology, University of Surrey.

'In the beginner's mind there are many possibilities. In the expert's mind there are few.'

Japanese proverb

'The reader's notes should be the outcome of understanding and not the prelude to it. Notes of this kind are brief.'

De Leeuw, M. and De Leeuw, E. (1991) *Read Better, Read Faster: A new approach to efficient reading.* London: Penguin Books.

Think about the process you go through when you make notes.

- What are its advantages?
- What are its shortcomings?
- How can you make the process work better?

Have an attempt at making a mind map. Read one of Tony Buzan's books on the subject before you start, such as:

Buzan, T. (1989) *Use Your Head.* London: BBC Books.

Understanding statistical information

Many people are tempted to miss out the statistics in the results section and go straight to the conclusions. This is a mistake, because it is not possible to judge the value of a study unless it is known whether the data have been interpreted fairly.

The basic principles of statistics are not particularly difficult to understand. The books listed below give relatively painless introductions to the subject. Even if you know very little about statistics, you can still be alert to ways in which they may be misused.

Are the figures genuine?

Very occasionally, researchers fabricate results, so that all the statistical analysis and theoretical work based on them is worthless. It is very difficult to detect this kind of fraud, which is why a few celebrated cases have gone unnoticed for years. Your suspicions may be raised if the calculations work out too neatly, or if you have doubts about the account of how the results were gathered. However, dishonesty among researchers is not common.

Results may also be invalidated by unconscious bias in the way they are collected.

Are the results interpreted fairly?

Some people can have a motive for interpreting their figures in a particular way. For example, a manager may want to show where savings can be made, while a trainer may want to demonstrate that further investment is needed. A biased conclusion is not usually based on false results, but on the selective way figures are interpreted.

A simple example of biased interpretation can occur in the choice of presenting an average as a mean, a median or a mode.

The mean is obtained by adding up all the results and dividing the total by the number of results. If you spent £3, £4, £8, £7 and £5 on a set of presents, you would divide the total (£27) by 5 and be able to say that the average cost of the gifts was £5.40. The mean is the most commonly used type of average. It can give a misleading impression as it can be distorted by one or two untypical results; for example, if one of the presents cost £45.

The median is the middle result if you arrange all the results in numerical order. In the example of the presents, the median would be £5. If you spent £45, instead of £8, on the most expensive

The following book has a useful section on quantitative analysis:

Polit, D.F. and Hungler, B.P. (1993) *Essentials of Nursing Research* (3rd edition). Philadelphia: J.B. Lippincott Company.

You will also find a readable and informative introduction to the subject in:

Rowntree, D. (1981) *Statistics Without Tears: A primer for non-mathematicians*. London: Penguin.

John Allen Paulos succeeds in presenting numbers and statistics in a very accessible way. See:

Paulos, J. A. (1991) *Beyond Numeracy*. London: Penguin.

Statistics and quantitative methods are covered in more detail in Section 4.

'The population of a large area of China was 28 million. Five years later it was 105 million. Very little of that increase was real; the great difference could be explained only by taking into account the purposes of the two enumerations and the way people would be inclined to feel about being counted in each instance. The first census was for tax and military purposes, the second for famine relief.'

Huff, D. (1954) *How to Lie with Statistics*. London: Victor Gollancz

Imagine you were the financial director of an organisation which employed a hundred poorly paid workers and four directors on very high salaries. The union representative comes to you to discuss a pay rise.

- Which type of average would you choose to describe the average pay within the organisation?
- Which type of average would the union representative be likely to use?

gift, the median would still be £5. It can be a useful type of average to use in situations where you have one or two extreme results.

The mode is the result which occurs most frequently. If someone asked you how long it usually took you to travel to work, you might think: 'If I catch the bus, which I usually do, it takes me half an hour. Of course, if I get a lift in, it will take less time and if I miss the bus and have to wait for the next bus it will take me 50 minutes. But most days I catch the bus, so the best answer is half an hour.' Here, you would be giving the mode.

Is the effect caused by chance?

Many research studies attempt to show a correlation between different variables, such as a relationship between people's age and their willingness to accept a new therapy. Statisticians do this by establishing that the effect is unlikely to have been caused by chance. Look for evidence that the researcher has subjected the results to a statistical test.

Have cause and effect been established?

Sometimes, a definite relationship can be found between different variables. But cause and effect may not have been established in the way the researcher claims. For example, a survey might reveal that smokers have lower salaries than non-smokers. Does this mean that smokers are less likely to be promoted, or that people smoke because they are undervalued at work, or that the smoking and the lower salaries are both influenced by another factor not mentioned in the survey, such as age or educational qualifications?

Has the researcher made a mistake in the analysis?

You need an extensive knowledge of statistics to check an analysis of results thoroughly. But some mistakes are surprisingly common. You may find examples where an attempt has been made to analyse figures which have no numerical meaning. This can happen where an ordinal scale, such as responses (from '0' very unfavourable to '7' very favourable) to an event are recorded. The numbers 0 to 7 cannot be used for calculations. They are simply convenient labels and the interval between them cannot be assumed to be equal.

Commonly used statistical tests:

- t-Test
- Median Test
- Mann-Whitney U Test
- Wilcoxon Signed-Rank Test
- Analysis of Variance (ANOVA)
- Chi-squared Test
- Pearson's Product-Moment Correlation
- Spearman's rho

You may find it interesting to collect examples of the misuse of statistics which appear in the national press. See the unit *Influences in Health Care: Media perspectives* for more on this issue.

The Ministry of Plenty's forecast had estimated the output of boots for the quarter at 145 million pairs. The actual output was given as sixty-two millions. Winston, however, in rewriting the forecast, marked the figure down to fifty-seven millions, so as to allow for the usual claim that the quota had been overfulfilled. In any case, sixty-two millions was no nearer the truth than fifty-seven millions, or than 145 millions. Very likely no boots had been produced at all. Likelier still, nobody knew how many had been produced, much less cared. All one knew was that every quarter astronomical numbers of boots were produced on paper, while perhaps half the population of Oceania went barefoot.'

Orwell, G. (1949) *Nineteen Eighty-Four*. London: Secker & Warburg.

Married men aged between 25 and 44 are statistically three times less likely to kill themselves than single, divorced and widowed men in the same age group.

How many theories can you think of which could explain this fact?

Conclusion

This Section has looked at how to conduct a literature search. As well as reading academic books and articles which are directly related to your research topic, be aware of other sources of information. Sometimes, you may have to go outside your own immediate field to find out about concepts or techniques which could contribute to your study. Other documents, such as policy statements, press reports and government statistics may also be relevant. What you discover as a result of the literature search should form the framework for the rest of your enquiry.

The Section also introduced some techniques for reading and taking notes. The most important thing you can do is to develop the habit of making reading an active process in which you engage critically with what the author is saying.

More suggestions for organising the information you gather in your literature search are given in Section 4. There is also some advice on the presentation of your review in Section 5.

'Academic knowledge involves two equally important elements: bodies of knowledge and methods of enquiry.'

Coben. D. and Hull, C. (1994) Professional training or academic education – a common problem? *Journal of Interprofessional Care* 8(1): 49.

A researcher writes:

'I think of reports like an onion – there are lots of layers. You keep adding them as you draft and re-draft. I suppose notes and jottings are the first layer, but the literature review is really the beginning. I always feel that the report is under way when I've done that bit.'

References

Hesse, M. (1980) *Revolutions and Reconstructions in the Philosophy of Science*. Brighton: Harvester.

Leedy, P. (1989) The review of related literature. In: Leedy, P. *Practical Research: Planning and design* (4th edition). New York: Macmillan.

O'Connor, S. E. (1992) Network theory - a systematic method for literature review. *Nurse Education Today* 12: 44-50.

Ryan, R. J., Scapens, R. W., and Theobald, M. (1991) *Research Methods and Methodologies in Accounting and Finance*. London: Academic Press.

Part of learning and reflection is recognising the learning processes that go on as you experience them. Here is a list of processes identified by an experienced adult educator:

- Maintain self-esteem and become increasingly responsible for learning and find direction for learning and invest energy in it
- Deal with personal energy ebb and flow
- Relate to others, but do find personal meaning in content and experiences
- Consolidate and synthesise new learning
- Test new ideas, skills, behaviour, ways of being
- Ask for and use feedback
- Plan how to use new learning in other situations
- Find and accept satisfactions, joys, excitement in learning.

Griffin, V. (1987) Naming the process. In: Boud, D. and Griffin, V. (eds). *Appreciating Adults Learning: From the learner's perspective.* London: Kogan Page.

Introduction

This Section takes you through the stages of the enquiry process. It:

- Describes the options you have at each stage
- Shows some of the implications of decisions you take
- Provides information about what is involved in various types of enquiry.

The Section starts with an overview of the enquiry process and describes some tools you can use to plan your own project.

You might want to read this Section at the same time as working on your own project. It will take you through the conceptual and data collection phases of your study to the point where you have analysed your results and decided your conclusions. Section 5 offers advice on writing up and presenting your research.

'Learning is not finding out what other people already know, but is solving our own problems for our own purposes, by questioning, thinking and testing until the solution is a new part of our life.'

Handy, C. (1989) The *Age of Unreason*. London: Arrow Books.

Enquiry is a way of understanding problems more deeply - and maybe even solving them. As you plan and carry out your enquiry, use your learning journal or diary to help you:

- Formulate the problem
- Think about how you are approaching it
- Test new information against your own purposes.

Educator Rudolph Flesch said that: 'Creative thinking may simply mean the realisation that there is no particular virtue in doing things the way they have always been done.'

Quoted in von Oech, R. (1990) *A Whack on the Side of the Head: How you can be more creative.* New York: Warner Books.

If it seems difficult or impossible to carry out your enquiry in the way you first thought, think of other possibilities. Talk with friends and colleagues, look at different approaches, think again. At this stage, be practical.

'Nursing is dynamic and interactive and it could be suggested that the rigorous academic approach to scientific research cannot appropriately integrate nursing theory and practice. A more reflexive approach involving a participative and collaborative style of research to bridge the theory/practice gap might be appropriate both for nursing and other professionals using practical skills.'

Green S. (1991) Weaving the web of knowledge. *The Health Service Journal* 101 (September 19): 22-23.

Overview of the enquiry process

There are three main phases in the process of enquiry:

- Conceptual phase - developing the research design
- Empirical phase - collecting your data
- Interpretative phase - analysing and interpreting your data.

The conceptual phase

Before starting this phase, you should have a good idea about:

- The different kinds of enquiry you might undertake
- The general subject of your project
- Which type of research is likely to be most appropriate.

In the conceptual phase, you will finalise these decisions. The literature review also forms part of this phase of the enquiry process (see Section 3 for ways of carrying out a literature review). Before going on to the next phase, you will have to decide which tools you are going to use to collect data and identify your sample.

The empirical phase

The empirical phase is the time of data collection. This process includes developing and testing the tools you are using for data collection. For example, if you are devising a questionnaire, you will need to pilot it on a few people first.

The interpretative phase

In the final phase you interpret the results, make your conclusions and recommendations and write up the study in a report. In some kinds of qualitative research, interpretation can start while the data are still being gathered.

'The History of every major Galactic Civilization tends to pass through three distinct and recognisable phases, those of Survival, Inquiry and Sophistication, otherwise known as the How, Why and Where phases.

For instance, the first phase is characterised by the question *How can we eat?* the second by the question *Why do we eat?* and the third by the question *Where shall we have lunch?*'

Adams, D. (1979) *The Hitch Hiker's Guide to the Galaxy*. London: Pan.

How do the activities in the box at the top of the opposite page relate to the three phases of a project?

Using the list on the opposite page as a guide, write a rough plan of what you think you will do to complete your project. At this point, many details may be unclear to you. But it is extremely useful to record:

- Decisions you are reasonably sure about
- Specific areas of knowledge you know you need to acquire
- Stages which are a complete mystery to you at the moment.

Work out a rough timescale for your activities. You will probably make changes to the outline plan as you get more deeply in to the project.

Planning the project

The list alongside shows the activities you will go through in the course of your enquiry-based project. For the sake of simplicity, a linear progression through the various stages is shown. In reality, you will probably find that you revisit some of these stages. For example:

- In the literature search you may find out about a new aspect of your subject which is potentially much more interesting and decide to reword your question
- When you begin to think in detail about research tools, you may find that your original research design is not practicable and that you have to rethink it.

Within the conceptual phase of a project, this kind of reassessment and adjustment is to be expected.

Pages 77-83 of this Section provide you with information and tools which should help you to plan your project.

- Decide the research question
- Carry out a literature search
- Choose a research design
- Choose the research tools
- Consider ethical issues
- If necessary, pilot the research
- Collect data
- Analyse data
- Interpret the results
- Draw conclusions
- Identify the limitations of the study
- Make recommendations
- Write up the research.

'The teacher's work, therefore, begins when that other person asks a question. No question, no teaching. But it is important to understand what a teacher can do and does with his answers, and what he cannot do. He does not give knowledge. Knowledge cannot be given. If you ask me a question all I can do in my reply is try to put into words a part of my experience. But you get only the words, not the experience. To make meaning out of my words, you must use your own experience.'

Holt, J. (1976) *Instead of Education: Ways to help people do things better.* London: Penguin.

Think about how you can best work with your tutor/counsellor to make the most of his/her experience.

In your learning journal, note down:

- What experience the tutor/counsellor put into words for you
- How you used your own experience to make meaning out of the tutor/counsellor's words.

As you work through the stages of your project, record your movements through the list above. Which stages do you have to revisit?

You may like to draw your own flow chart as you progress. It could include arrows showing when you returned to an earlier stage.

'Research is a process. It starts with a puzzle; proceeds to a literature or knowledge review; and goes on to the specification of an answerable question; the design of an appropriate methodology; the collection of appropriate information; and the analysis of information, and its dissemination to interested colleagues.'

Brooks, N. (1988) Why research? *British Journal of Occupational Therapy* 51(11): 397-98.

Getting the scale right

Until you have had personal experience of doing research, it can be difficult to know how much time it takes to complete the various tasks involved. As a result, some students attempt projects which are too ambitious and are disappointed when they have to change plans to get their work finished on time.

On these two pages you will find some advice from experienced researchers which may help you to decide an appropriate scale for your project. The times given here can only be approximate - you may work faster or slower - but they should provide you with some useful rules of thumb.

Interviews

If you are going to analyse unstructured interviews, you need to transcribe them word for word. Allow between eight to 12 hours to transcribe a one-hour interview, unless you are a very experienced audio typist. The process of coding an interview of this length will probably take you between two and three hours. Three one-hour unstructured interviews may be an acceptable minimum on which to base your project, but get advice from your tutor/counsellor.

Structured interviews are much quicker to analyse, but you are likely to need more of them. You can listen to the tape and fill in a coding sheet as you go, only pausing to transcribe key sections.

Questionnaires

Many people make their questionnaires too long, which reduces the response rate and makes them harder to analyse. Aim for a maximum total of 30 questions - many fewer may give you all the information you want. A response rate of between 50 and 60% for a questionnaire is good, but this may be increased if you can find some way of motivating people to complete it.

If you write the questionnaire yourself, it will probably take you about five or six hours to prepare a first draft. Then allow time to pilot and rewrite it and re-pilot it. It is relatively quick to code questionnaires. It will probably take you about four to six hours to code 50 questionnaires.

Observation

Allow time to visit the setting and become accepted by the people you will be observing before you start gathering data. You may need to

'All too often people embark on research projects without sufficient consideration of the time they will take and assume that it is possible to do a normal day's work and squeeze research in too. When time is short, patient care takes priority over research and if hospital workers are already burdened, the knowledge that research findings may ultimately benefit this care is of little consequence.'

Green S. (1991) Weaving the web of knowledge. *The Health Service Journal* 101 (September 19): 22-23.

'Many of us pay lip service to the need for this type of rigour but dislike abiding by the rules...particularly when it involves working four nights a week driving around council estates in the dark and the rain. Such an approach is, however, essential if we are to produce results that are reliable, valid and sensitive.'

Goble, R. (1989) Research in occupational therapy: luxury or necessity? *British Journal of Occupational Therapy* 52(9): 349-51.

Talk to other researchers and find out where they had difficulties.

Don't forget your other commitments and build in some time for the unforeseeable.

The section of a research report which describes the limitations of the study can often be extremely illuminating for other researchers. Learn from the difficulties of others and, when it comes to your own report, be honest about the problems which you faced.

do more than one 'dummy run'. It generally takes less time to be accepted as a non-participant observer than as a participant observer.

Field notes

If the research is based on observation, write up field notes as soon as possible. Remember to leave time for this or you will lose a lot of valuable information. If you plan to observe a situation for an hour, arrange to have another hour immediately afterwards in which you can write up your notes.

Literature search

Allow time to:
- Identify the texts
- Obtain copies of the texts
- Read them.

If your library is equipped with an electronic database, a few hours may be enough to identify the key texts, although you will almost certainly have to return later to check other references. When it comes to obtaining texts which your library does not hold, you are at the mercy of the administrative system used to borrow books from other collections. It is best to discuss this with your librarian at an early stage.

The speed at which you read will be personal to you. You will probably get quicker as you become more familiar with the subject matter.

Writing up your project

Allow a week of full-time work, about 40 hours, to write up your project. This assumes that you have already been through the process of writing it up in draft form - and you may have several drafts. Some people will take considerably longer than this.

If you can, give yourself some leeway here, so that if you do run into difficulties at this last stage you are still able to do justice to the work you have put in earlier. Also, leave time for proof-reading, copying, final checking and binding.

How much time do you have?

Make a realistic assessment of the time you actually have available to work on your project. Most people also have other demands on their time and and energy.

	Mon	Tues	Wed	Thur	Fri	Sat	Sun
00							
01							
02							
03							
04							
05							
06							
07							
08							
09							
10							
11							

It can be useful to look at your working, sleeping and studying patterns over a week, using an hour-by-hour chart, like this.

If you haven't already done so, think carefully about what time you are able to devote to your project each week.

It might be helpful to draw up a chart similar to that alongside this text showing the 24 hours in each day of the week. Block out the time you need to sleep and spend on other commitments. Decide how much of the rest of the time you can give to your project work. Be realistic about it, and don't devise a plan that will leave you exhausted.

Monitor yourself for a week or two. Don't worry if you don't keep exactly to your schedule, but examine why you didn't.

Managing your project

Project management techniques can help you to make the best use of resources as you carry out your project. The next four pages describe tools which could be useful for project planning.

Flowcharts

A flowchart is a diagram which shows the operations which make up a process. It can also indicate alternative courses of action following decisions. A flowchart can help you:

- Check that you really understand the process
- Think about the implications for time and other resources of any decisions that have to be made along the way
- Simplify and streamline the process.

Critical path analysis

This is a technique used in project management when a number of different tasks are going on at the same time. Critical path analysis is a very good way of working out the most logical order of doing things and of planning realistic schedules. The following simple example, based on photocopying a questionnaire and inserting it in envelopes for posting, will show you how the technique works.

1. Start by listing all the tasks.
2. Some tasks can't start until others have been completed. Arrange the tasks in a logical order.

As Fig 1. shows, some of the tasks can be done at the same time.

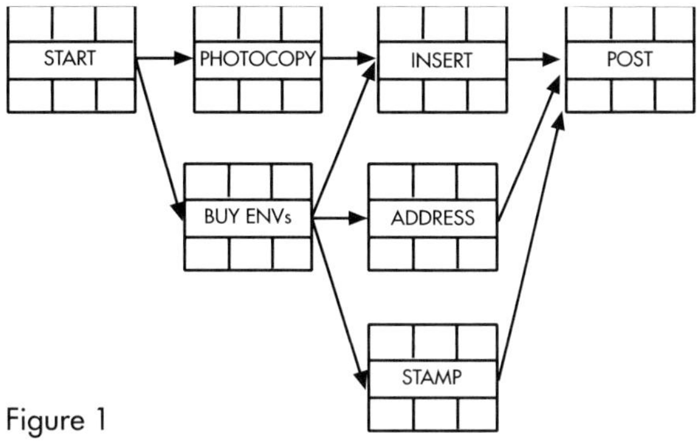

Figure 1

3. Fill in the duration time of each task (See Figure 2). In the worked examples (Figs 3-5), the time is shown in minutes.

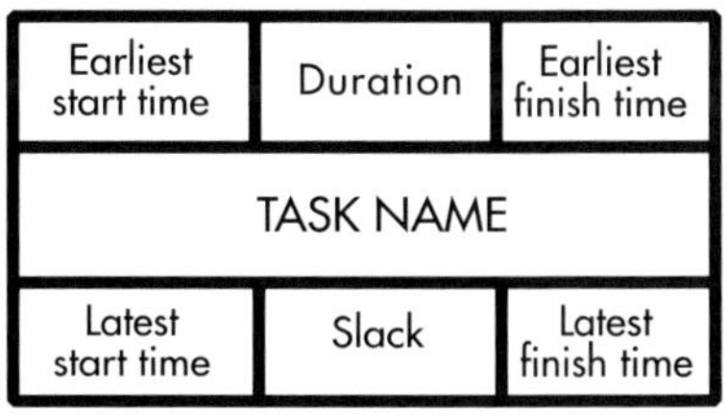

Figure 2

4. Work through Figure 3 from the left and calculate the earliest start and finishing time for each task.

Draw a flowchart to show the process you use when following up a reference and locating an article in a research journal.

Could you simplify the process?

In the example described above, some tasks are going on simultaneously. This means that two people would be required to complete the process in the minimum time. When you are doing your project, you will probably be working alone most of the time. But there may be times when other people are working on your behalf, for example by piloting your questionnaire or responding to requests for information.

The flowchart on the opposite page shows the process of approaching a random sample of staff with children and asking them to complete a questionnaire. As you can see, the researcher first establishes whether the member of staff is part of the population under study (staff with children) and then asks him or her to participate in the survey. The process is repeated until the researcher has enough potential respondents.

The symbol (a) indicates a stage in the process:

(a) 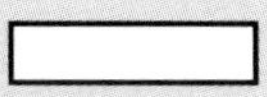

The symbol (b) indicates a decision:

(b) 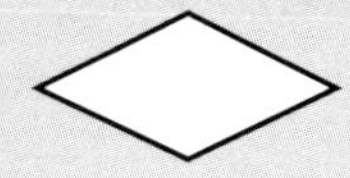

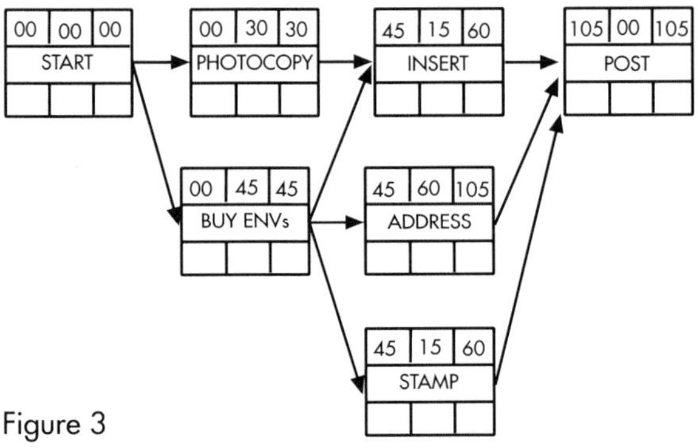

Figure 3

5. Now work out the latest time each task can start and finish (Figure 4).

6. Fill in the 'slack' by deducting the earliest start time from the latest start time in each box (Figure 5).

The critical path is the one which passes through the boxes with no slack. If these tasks are delayed, the whole project will be late, so this is where you have to concentrate your efforts. You can be more flexible with tasks which have a lot of slack and do them when it is most convenient.

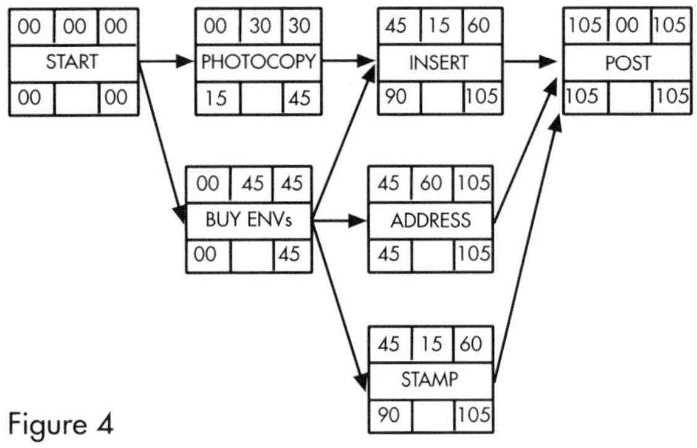

Figure 4

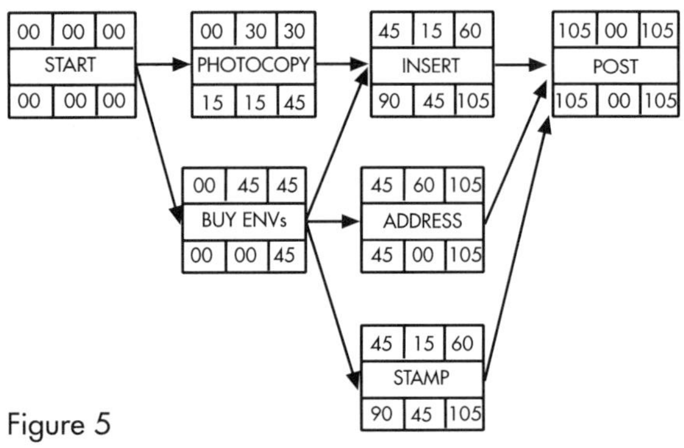

Figure 5

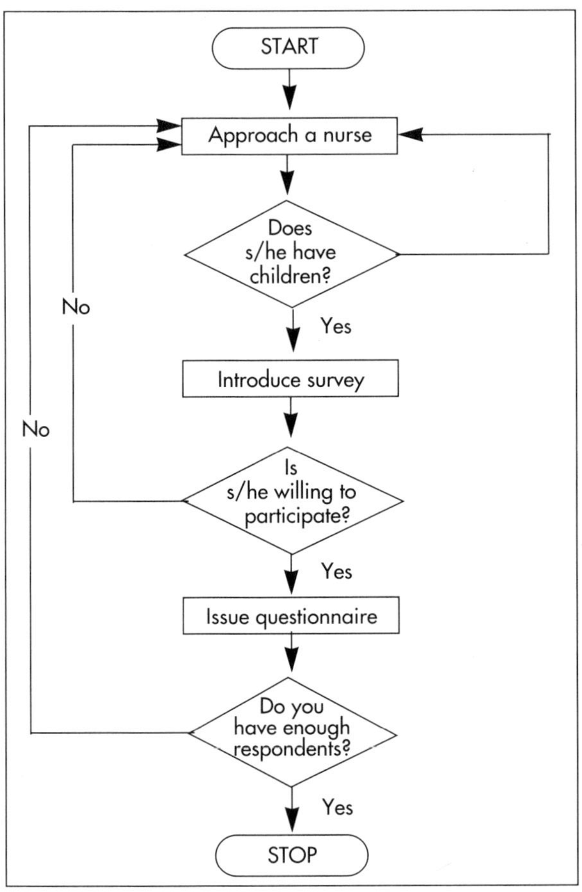

What would happen to the overall timing of the process described in the diagrams above if it actually took half an hour (not 15 minutes) to insert the envelopes?

What would happen if it took an hour to go and buy the envelopes?

Try using critical path analysis to work out how you will organise a self-contained part of your project, such as the literature search.

Are there times in your project where you think you will have several tasks going on at once? Would it be helpful to analyse them using critical path analysis?

More planning tools

When you know what tasks you have to do and the order in which they have to be done, you need to plan a schedule. A Gantt chart is a useful technique to use for this. This is a chart which shows activities, usually represented by bars or horizontal lines, in a timeframe. It allows you to see at a glance how things are going. Gantt charts are often used when a series of stages are repeated, perhaps on different batches of material.

You have almost certainly seen charts of this kind in a work setting. Many variations are possible. You can add symbols for key events and also include a projected and actual schedule on the same grid. Colour coding is often used.

A Gantt chart makes clear the implications of any delay in part of the process. If one stage takes longer than anticipated, all the following stages will have to be moved up the grid as well. For this reason, it is useful if the chart is prepared in a form that can be updated. Special laminated charts are available, or you can draw up your grid on ordinary paper and make several copies. The best solution is to use scheduling or project management software, to make the updating easy. A Gantt chart should be displayed prominently so that it can be a constant reminder of priorities.

Looking at cause and effect

Another planning tool that you may find useful is the fishbone diagram. This lists possible causes for an observed effect. It could be helpful if you were considering rival hypotheses or planning the information it would be relevant to gather in a questionnaire.

Follow these stages:

- Write the effect in a box on the right
- On a separate piece of paper, think of as many causes of this effect as you can
- Group the effects into different categories, such as 'staff attitudes', 'skills and knowledge', 'resources', 'patient's attitudes', or whatever is appropriate to the situation you are looking at
- Add the causes to the branches of the diagram.

A fishbone diagram gives you an overall picture of a situation and helps you decide where to focus your attention.

Two techniques which may be useful when you are making decisions are decision boxes and decision trees

Think about if it would be useful to draw up a Gantt chart for your project. Take a critical look at the charts used in your workplace to explain schedules.

Are there any techniques you could usefully adapt for your own purposes?

This simple Gantt chart shows a schedule for observing and interviewing participants at two different sites. The figures refer to weeks. How would the chart have to be changed if the observation at the first site was delayed until the second week?

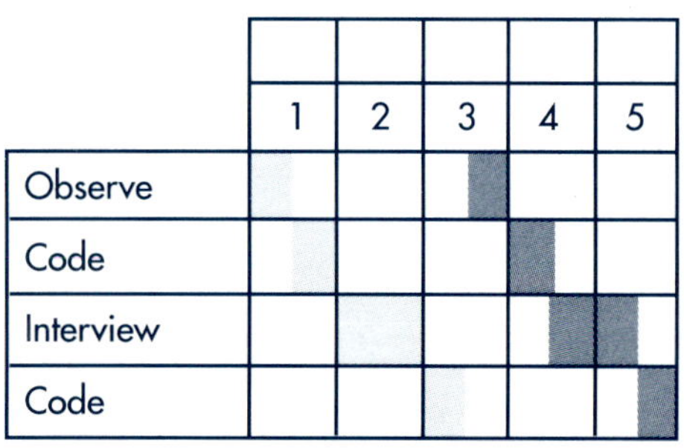

The fishbone diagram below analyses possible causes for the low take-up of smoking cessation classes at a GP's surgery. What lines of research does it suggest to you?

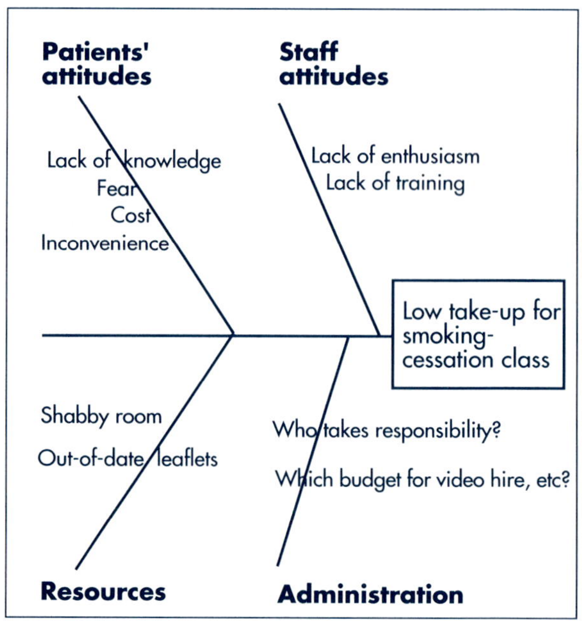

Decision boxes

Write the decision in a box in the middle of a piece of paper (see box below). On the left, list all the reasons for making this decision. On the right, list the reasons against it. You can then evaluate the reasons and make your decision. This method is helpful when you need to verbalise your real concerns.

Decision trees

It is sometimes helpful to break a decision down into several smaller decisions. This can be done by drawing a decision tree, like the example shown opposite. In certain circumstances you may be able to estimate the consequences of each choice, which will aid the decision-making process. In other situations, the act of drawing a decision tree will simply help clarify your logic and enable you to explain and justify your decision in your report.

Example of a decision tree to observe the behaviour of receptionists dealing with patients

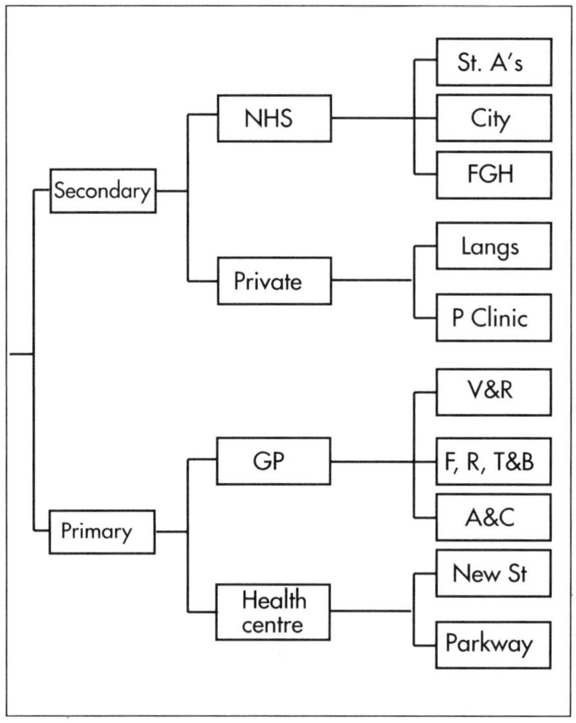

Example of a decision box

For		Against
Accuracy	Tape-record the interviews	Could intimidate people
Quicker than making notes		
Can concentrate on noting non-verbal behaviour		Lack of frankness
Accepted research procedure		The technology could make me nervous
Better eye contact		

Look at the decision box above.

- What do you think was the real concern of the researcher who drew up this chart?
- Would you add any more reasons for or against tape-recording interviews in your research?
- What would you decide to do?

The decision tree above was drawn up by a researcher who was trying to select sites where she could observe the behaviour of receptionists dealing with patients.

Prepare a decision tree to choose your research design.

Stating the problem

Before you start your project, you should state clearly the problem you are addressing. If you have worked through Section 1, you probably will have already identified the issue you want to study and started to clarify the scope of your investigations.

The convention is to write a problem for enquiry either as a statement or a question. For example:

- The purpose of this project is to investigate the relationship between female midwives' personal experiences of labour and their attitude to women in the delivery room.
- What is the relationship between female midwives' personal experiences of labour and their attitude to women in the delivery room?

Your problem should state the key study variables, which you must be able to measure or observe, and indicate the population to be studied. In the above example, the key variables are 'the experience of labour' and 'the attitude to women in the delivery room'. The population to be studied is 'female midwives'.

Notice that this is not 'female midwives who have had children', as the experience of midwives who have no personal knowledge of childbirth will also contribute to the study. The problem could be studied by interviewing midwives about their experiences of labour and their attitude to women in the delivery room - it might be difficult actually to observe their behaviour in the delivery room. In order to do this, you would need permission from the women, the staff and the managers of the unit. You may also have to obtain clearance from the ethics committee.

You may have to adjust the problem in the conceptual phase of the enquiry. One reason to do this would be if a literature search revealed other, more potentially valuable, lines of enquiry or perhaps made you aware of problems faced by earlier researchers that you had not considered.

If you discovered that exactly the same problem had been investigated in previous research, this would not necessarily be a reason to abandon your own project. Replication studies make a useful contribution to research. But in this case, you should make it an explicit part of your project to examine how far your own investigations confirmed or called into question the earlier study.

'Just before she died she asked: "What is the answer?" No answer came. She laughed aloud and said: "In that case, what is the question?" Then she died.'

The last words of Gertrude Stein quoted in Sutherland, D. (1951) *Gertrude Stein: A biography of her work.* Connecticut: Yale University Press.

Write down the problem you will be addressing in your own enquiry-based project.

- What are the key study variables?
- How will you observe or measure them?
- What is the population?

'Questions are the engines of intellect, the cerebral machines which convert . . . curiosity to controlled enquiry.' Fischer, D. H. (1970) *Historians' Fallacies: Toward a logic of historical thought.* New York: Harper Torchbooks.

Check your stated problem against these questions:

- Am I genuinely interested in this topic?
- Whom will it benefit?
- Will it help improve practice? How?
- Will it help develop theory? How?
- Do I have the resources to do it?
- What support from other people do I need, and am I likely to get it?
- Do I have relevant knowledge and experience?
- Is the investigation ethically acceptable?

'When I use a word', Humpty Dumpty said, in a rather scornful tone, 'it means just what I choose it to mean — neither more nor less.'

Carroll, L. (1970) *The Annotated Alice: Alice's Adventures in Wonderland* and *Through the Looking Glass.* London: Penguin.

Think about how the use of key words may shape your approach to the topic.

Research hypotheses

You may be able to base your study around a research hypothesis. This is a statement of the predicted relationship between two or more variables. In the example discussed here, a possible hypothesis could be:

- Female midwives who have had a difficult experience of labour themselves are more likely than those who have not had such an experience to empathise with women in the delivery room.

A hypothesis needs to:

- Be written in a declarative sentence - a statement, not a question
- Include the population
- Include the variables
- Reflect the problem to be addressed in the enquiry
- Be empirically testable.

Hypotheses can be described as simple or complex. A simple hypothesis contains one independent and one dependent variable. A complex hypothesis contains two or more independent variables, two or more dependent variables, or both.

The way to test a hypothesis is to gather data which, after statistical analysis, will either support or fail to support it. A hypothesis cannot be said to be proved or disproved. The process of testing a research hypothesis involves stating an alternative 'null hypothesis' which states that there is no significant relationship between the variables. This can then be statistically tested. If the analysis of data does not support the null hypothesis, then the research hypothesis is supported.

A non-directional hypothesis suggests that there is a relationship between the variables, but does not specify what it is. A directional hypothesis goes further and states the type of relationship that you expect to find. A directional hypothesis should be based on existing theory.

A hypothesis is appropriate only in the type of enquiry where enough is known about the topic to make a reasonable prediction. The data gathered must also be capable of statistical analysis.

Read these two hypotheses:

- Birth weight is lower among infants of alcoholic mothers than among infants of non-alcoholic mothers
- Daily weight loss is greater for adults who follow a reduced calorie diet and exercise daily than for those who do not follow a reduced calorie diet and do not exercise daily.

Can you identify:

- The population?
- The independent variable?
- The dependent variable?

Would you describe these as simple or complex?

Is it appropriate to base your research around a hypothesis?

If so, write it down and state:

- The population
- The independent variable
- The dependent variable
- How you will test it
- Whether your hypothesis is simple or complex.

Think about the meanings of the following words. Using them might help you approach and refine your research topic:

- Analyse
- Argue
- Compare
- Criticise
- Define
- Describe
- Discuss
- Enumerate
- Evaluate
- Examine
- Trace
- Explain
- Illustrate
- Interpret
- Justify
- Outline
- Prove
- Relate
- Review
- State
- Summarise

Organising a literature review

The conventional time to undertake a literature review is at the start of a project, when you are still deciding the problem to be addressed and the way you will design your enquiry. Doing it at the start means that these important decisions will be informed by the work of other people in the area.

In her description of how she formulated her research problem on informal care of people with dementia, Taraborrelli (1992) outlined how a review of the literature revealed much useful information about informal care. She found material dealing with the economic, social and psychological costs of informal care and on the social foundations of informal care. What was missing was a conceptualisation of how the carer's role may change over time. She found a useful model for this in a study which examined the process of becoming a professional carer, based on how medical students become doctors.

There is one type of research — grounded theory — where you should delay looking at the literature until you have gathered your data.

Grounded theory is an ethnographic form of research in which theories are obtained from the data itself and not from the researcher's previous knowledge or understanding of the subject. In these circumstances, a review of the literature could distort the researcher's initial perceptions. But in most types of enquiry, an early review of the literature is regarded as essential.

Your literature search can reveal:

- Classic studies on the same or similar topics
- Underlying theories which should inform analysis of the concepts you are dealing with
- Background information, such as official statistics on the prevalence of a problem
- Information on methodology and statistical analysis
- Specific tools, such as existing questionnaires or interview guides, which you could use in your own enquiry.

Guidance on how to go about a literature search is given in Section 3. If you are very lucky, you may be able to identify most of the important literature in the first round of your search, but it is more likely that the books and articles you read will provide references to other material. You may also become aware of gaps in the literature which you may be able to fill by using the literature of allied disciplines.

> In a private debate the scholar Salih Awami said to Sufi Rahimi:
>
> 'What you have just said lacks references and proofs through quotations from ancient authority.'
>
> 'Not at all', said Rahimi, 'for I have them all here, chapter and verse.'
>
> The scholar went away saying, 'That was what I wanted to know.'
>
> The next day he made his famous speech on Rahimi which began:
>
> 'The lecture which you are about to hear from Sheikh Rahimi lacks conviction. Why, he is so unsure of himself that he actually adduced written proofs and authorities to what he says'.
>
> Shah, I. (1974) Rahimi. In: *Thinkers of the East.* London: Penguin.

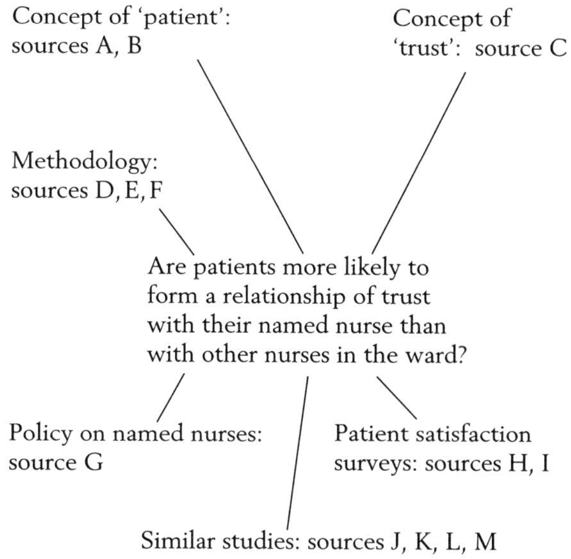

> Draw a diagram showing what sources you have used to explore different aspects of the problem you are addressing. Are there any gaps? If so, how will you fill them?

When you come to present your literature review, your assessor will be looking for evidence that you have:

- Described material that is relevant to your research topic
- Covered all essential aspects of the research problem in your review
- Been critical in your reading
- Understood the implications of what you have read for your own research
- Taken note of studies where the conclusions contradict your own work
- Used material that is up to date.

How to organise your notes

These suggestions are adapted from Leedy (1989):

- Write your problem at the top of the page where you cannot lose sight of it. It is the central axis around which everything else revolves.
- Dissect the problem by numbering and naming its various sub-parts.
- Note the particular sub-division of the problem to which the study relates, and the rationale for including it in the review of the literature
- Gather together all the citations that refer to a particular aspect of the problem, so that you have as many groups as you have sub-divisions of your main problem
- Study these groups in relation to each other, with a view to planning and organising the discussion of the related literature
- Write the review. Head each section with headings, whose wording contains the identical words found in the statement of the problem.

When you have completed a literature review, ask yourself these questions:

- How has the literature reviewed contributed to your understanding of the research question?
- What procedures did you use to gather the literature?
- Were they successful?
- If not, what else should you have done?

Here are some typical criticisms of the material discussed in literature reviews. Could they be levelled at you?

- The works listed are secondary sources, not the original research studies themselves.
- The literature is out of date and does not reflect modern thinking in this area.
- The literature is only peripherally relevant to the topic of the research.

One student says:

'As I was often in a rush, I used to neglect to note minor details like date and place of publication. To my cost, I learned how much time can be wasted having to go back and find the references. Now I make a note of absolutely all the information I might need.'

Time spent keeping track of references as you carry our your literature search will save much heartache later on. There are several different forms of referencing, the most common of which is the Harvard system, used in this book.

'Education . . . has produced a vast population able to read but unable to distinguish what is worth reading. . .

Trevelyan, G. M. (1948) *English Social History*. London: The Reprint Society.

Remember to evaluate your selected material on the basis of the purpose for which you need it.

Designing the study

The way you design a project is closely linked to the choice of problem. In deciding the problem you have already gone a long way towards deciding the type of enquiry you will undertake.

Use these two pages to check:
- Which type of enquiry method is most appropriate for your problem
- Whether it is practicable to undertake this type of enquiry
- Whether you are comfortable with the implications of your choice of problem.

What is appropriate to the topic?

A quantitative study measures relationships between variables. A qualitative study is concerned with exploring concepts, situations and attitudes. If your topic is one for which a great deal of exploratory work has been done, you may feel that the time has come to test out some of these theories in a quantitative study — a literature review will reveal the current state of knowledge on your topic.

However, if little has been written about your topic of enquiry, you are aware of gaps in this work, or you disagree with its conceptual basis, a qualitative study may be more appropriate.

Many topics are first researched in qualitative studies then followed up, often by different researchers with other skills and interests, in quantitative research. Sometimes it happens the other way round. For example, a quantitative study could establish that a relationship exists between a patient's age and willingness or reluctance to be seen by a practice nurse instead of a GP. A qualitative study could examine why this relationship existed.

Section 2 outlined the different types of qualitative research. Very broadly:
- *Ethnography*: looks at how individuals within a particular society view the world
- *Phenomenology*: attempts to capture the actual experience of being in a situation
- *Emancipatory research*: is concerned with using knowledge to empower individuals

Ethnographic studies are usually based on a combination of interviews and observation, which are then subjected to analysis. A phenomenological study could use unstructured interviews with participants, or gather data from diaries, life stories, newspapers, films or poetry. One of the

Ideas about what can and cannot be measured change over time. This is how the quantitative methods of Harvey, who discovered the circulation of the blood, were criticised by a contemporary:

'Of a truth, you do not use your eyes or command them to be used, but instead rely on reasoning and calculation, reckoning at carefully selected moments how many pounds of blood, how many ounces, how many drachms have to be transferred from the heart into the arteries in the space of one little half-hour. Truly, Harvey, you are pursuing a fact which cannot be investigated, a thing which is incalculable, inexplicable, unknowable.'

Quoted in: Boorstin D.J. (1984) *The Discoverers*. London: J.M. Dent & Sons Ltd.

Benoliel (1984) has identified the following four broad areas in which unstructured, qualitative approaches appear most promising:

- Environmental influences on care-giving systems
- Decision-making processes
- People's adaption to critical life experiences, such as chronic illness or developmental changes
- The nature of the nurse-client social transactions in relation to stability and change.'

Benoliel, J.Q. (1984) Advancing nursing science: qualitative approaches. *Western Journal of Nursing Research* 6:1-8.

Does your own research problem fall into one of these categories?

major characteristics of phenomenology is the fact that the meaning emerges from the participants in the phenomenon and is not imposed by the researcher. In emancipatory research, the relationship between the researcher and the participants in the research is different from that in the other paradigms: instead of distancing yourself as a researcher, your aim is to work with participants to make practical changes with your co-researchers or in your own personal practice.

Is it practicable?

In quantitative research, data are gathered and analysed from a large number of subjects or situations. In qualitative research, a smaller volume of subjects or situations is looked at in much more detail. Quantitative data are usually presented in a standard format, such as replies to a questionnaire, and are therefore relatively easy to manage. A qualitative study may have a large amount of data resulting from a small number of interviews or observations.

A small quantitative study is unlikely to have statistical value. A small qualitative study can still yield useful information, because it does not depend for its value on the generalisability of its conclusions. If you have very limited time available for your project, a qualitative study may be your only realistic option.

Think about what kind of access you have to potential participants. It is usually not possible to do research work on patients or clients without clearance from an ethical committee. There may also be a local policy of discouraging students from working with patients. If you are interested in emancipatory research, consider whether you will need, and be given, permission to carry it out in your workplace.

Your own skills and preferences

All data, however gathered, need to be analysed. If you undertake a survey, conventional statistical methods should be used in the analysis. Software and statisticians can help you in this, but you do have to be systematic.

The further you move from quantitative research through ethnography and phenomenology towards emancipatory research, the more important your relationship with the participants becomes and the less you are able to rely on standardised methods of collecting and analysing data.

After reading these two pages, do you have any doubts about your research question and its implications for the kind of research you will undertake?

If so, consider them carefully before proceeding and, if necessary, rethink your research problem. You might find one of the decision-making tools on pages 82 and 83 useful here.

Take this opportunity to find out more about your chosen research design – perhaps by following up some of the references on pages 48 to 51.

Think about the following question if you plan to use observation techniques in your project:

- Would you enjoy the experience of observing your own colleagues at work?
- What difficulties can you anticipate?
- Would you feel more, or less, comfortable as an observer in a situation where you were not known personally?

For a description of what it is like to be a participant observer, read:

Wax, R.H. (1971) *Doing Fieldwork: Warnings and advice*. Chicago: University of Chicago Press.

Samples

When you undertake an enquiry, you identify the population to which the study applies. This population is the total of all the individuals or objects which share particular characteristics. For example, a population might be 'dietitians' or 'dietitians caring for people with diabetes'. It is usually impossible to study all members of a population and better to select a sample.

In quantitative research, the most important criterion when selecting a sample is the extent to which it is representative of the population. In qualitative research, generalisability of the results is not an issue, so it is not so important that the sample should be representative.

There are two approaches to sampling:

- Probability sampling
- Non-probability sampling.

Probability sampling

This is the more rigorous of the two approaches because it relies on random selection of the population. Each element (member of the population) has an equal, independent chance of being selected. This does not guarantee that the sample is representative, but it means that there are no other factors, apart from chance, that are interfering with the representativeness of the sample. The larger the sample is, the more likely it is to be representative. There are four commonly used designs for probability sampling.

1. *Simple random sampling:* every member of the population has an equal chance of being selected. To make a selection, you must have a list of all members of the population, known as a 'population frame'. Individuals are then picked at random from this list, using the technique described in the box below. For some populations, it is relatively easy to acquire a population frame. If you were studying the healthcare professionals employed by a particular health authority, you would probably be able to obtain a list. But it would be very difficult to obtain a list of 'all healthcare professionals in Scotland with children'. Problems associated with obtaining the population frame and then numbering all the individuals on it make simple random sampling impracticable in many situations.

2. *Systematic sampling:* this is a variation in which every 'nth' individual is chosen. You work out the value of 'n' by dividing the size of the population by the size of the sample you need.

> Think about how you could go about establishing a population frame for healthcare professionals in a particular setting.

> In simple random sampling, it is sometimes necessary to use existing lists as the population frame. The choice of list defines the population.
>
> If you used a telephone directory as a population frame, how would you define your population?

How to select a simple random sample

1. Start by establishing the population frame, identifying and defining a population.
2. Number the individuals on the list consecutively.
3. Using a table of random numbers, point with a pencil to a number on the table.
4. Move in a systematic way - up, down or diagonally - choosing a sample by picking those subjects whose numbers correspond to the table of random numbers.
5. Ignore numbers that do not appear on the frame (list).
6. Once a number is selected and becomes part of the sample, ignore it if it appears again.
7. Stop when the sample size is obtained.

You then pick a random number to identify the first individual from the population frame and count on 'n' in the list to identify the second, and so on.

3. *Stratified random sampling:* the population is first divided into two or more strata or sub-groups, with the aim of providing a more representative sample. For example, if the proportion of women to men in a population is in the ratio 60:40, this proportion of 60:40 is reflected in your sample. The selection is made by a similar method to a simple random sample.

4. *Cluster sampling*: the population is gathered into groups, or clusters. This method is often used with large-scale studies. Clusters are convenient groupings such as individual streets or districts and must themselves be randomly chosen from a population containing all streets or districts.

Non-probability sampling

This approach is unlikely to produce a representative sample. The methods described here are unsuitable for quantitative studies but can be used in qualitative research.

1. *Accidental sampling (also known as convenience sampling)*: the most convenient individuals for a sample are selected. For example a questionnaire might be handed out to the first 100 people to enter a building. This is a weak form of sampling because the available subjects may not be typical of the population as a whole.

2. *Quota sampling* : this is similar to stratified random sampling. The researcher builds in representativeness in the sample by mirroring characteristics of the population, such as age, gender or years of experience. Within these groups, accidental sampling is used.

3. *Purposive or judgement sampling* : the researcher makes the selection based on a judgment of who would be representative. This method is not recommended for quantitative studies, but is appropriate for qualitative research.

4. *Snowball sampling* : sometimes used when subjects are difficult to identify. One subject suggests other potential subjects and the sample grows (snowballs). It will not produce a representative sample, but may be a way of gaining access to subjects who are not listed anywhere - for example, people who have experienced faith healing.

Think about the sampling methods described on these two pages.

- What 'clusters' could you use if you were sampling healthcare professionals employed by a health authority?
- If you wanted to sample nurses in a hospital, why might you not get a representative sample if you selected every 10th nurse who walked into the canteen?

Can you think of any groups where snowball sampling might be the only method to obtain a sample?

Which method will you use to obtain the sample of your enquiry?

Gathering data – 1

These four pages look at the most common ways of gathering data from people:

- Questionnaires
- Interviews - structured, semi-structured or unstructured
- Observation.

Questionnaires

A questionnaire is a written set of questions which respondents answer themselves. Questions can be 'open', where respondents can answer in any way they like, or 'closed', where respondents choose from a limited set of answers. Open questions are difficult to analyse, but can provide more information.

Closed questions can take several forms:

- Dichotomous questions offer only two answers, usually 'yes' or 'no'
- Multiple-choice questions offer a wider range of responses, such as 'excellent, good, poor, extremely poor'
- 'Cafeteria' questions offer a range of answers, such as a range of statements from which respondents are asked to pick the one which most nearly corresponds to their own views
- Priority statements ask respondents to assign a priority to a set of alternatives, usually by writing numbers in boxes. They are useful for finding out which issues people feel most strongly about.

Respondents may be unwilling to give their own views in a questionnaire. One way round this is to ask an indirect question. Instead of asking 'What do you feel about the new ward procedure?', you could ask 'What do you think the general feeling is about the new ward procedure?' People appear to be comfortable expressing negative opinions if they can attribute them to others.

Questionnaires are a relatively cheap way of gathering large amounts of data. But they do demand very careful design and piloting, and may have a low response rate. If questionnaires are being filled in away from the setting to which they refer, as they might be if you were asking patients about their attitudes to waiting arrangements in a clinic, other factors might influence the answers. For example, patients might forget their irritation and discomfort once they had seen the doctor. Their response to the whole experience of visiting the clinic might be coloured by their experience in the consulting room.

If you are going to design your own questionnaire, an excellent handbook is:

Oppenheim, A.N. (1992) *Questionnaire Design and Attitude Measurement.* Aldershot: Gower.

A good source of information on surveys is:

Moser, C. and Kalton, G. (1971 *Survey Methods in Social Investigation.* Aldershot: Gower.

There is also a very useful section in:

Polit, D.F. and Hungler, B.P. (1993) *Essentials of Nursing Research* (3rd ed.) Philadelphia: J.B. Lippincott Company.

You could also consult:

Munn, P. and Drever, E. (1995) *Using Questionnaires in Small-scale Research: A teacher's guide* (revised edition) Edinburgh: Scottish Council for Research in Education.

When you are designing a questionnaire, why do you think it is often a good idea to ask about non-contentious issues first?

Try writing different types of question to discover healthcare professionals' attitudes about their personal safety at work. Write one or two of each type and try them out on your colleagues to see what sorts of answers they give. The different types are:

- Dichotomous
- Multiple-choice
- Cafeteria
- Priority
- Indirect.

If you are writing a questionnaire for your enquiry, include a variety of different questions.

Imagine you are sending out a questionnaire by post to people who work in a particular healthcare unit. How could you encourage your respondents to answer the questions truthfully and accurately?

Interviews

An interview is a face-to-face or telephone conversation between the researcher and respondent. Interviews can be structured to varying degrees.

A structured interview is similar to a questionnaire — the same questions are asked in the same order and in exactly the same way. Although it is time-consuming to interview people, the response rate is likely to be higher and it is easier to gain access to groups such as visually impaired people or children who would not be able to fill in a form themselves.

In a semi-structured interview, the same basic questions are asked, but the interviewer can vary the order and probe for more information. This can be useful if people need some help in understanding the questions, but the data obtained from a semi-structured interview are more difficult to analyse. The technique also requires more skill from the interviewer, so as to avoid leading the respondents to answer in a particular way.

In an unstructured interview, the interviewer goes in with a list of topics to cover, known as an 'interview guide' and is free to discuss them in any way. An unstructured interview is close to an ordinary conversation except that it is guided along pre-set lines by the researcher.

One way to prepare an interview guide is to think about the topic and write down as many things as possible that you would like to know about it. If you talk to other people and ask them what is interesting about the topic, you can add their perspectives, too. Next you sort the questions into themes and take a list of them into the interview. If you go through this process, you tend to remember the actual questions at the appropriate moments, and the flow of conversation is not broken up by your constantly looking at a list of questions.

Special methods are needed to analyse the data from an unstructured interview. The researcher has to look for patterns in the responses and find a way to code them (see pages 102-105).
When gathering data from interviews and observations, it is important not to forget demographic and other information about subjects, for example, age, occupation. Without this, it may be impossible to analyse the data in a meaningful way.

Watch a political interview on the television.

- What techniques does the interviewer use to ask probing questions?
- Would these techniques be appropriate in a research interview?
- How does the interviewee try to avoid answering difficult questions?
- Have you seen these techniques used in other situations?

You can find an interesting introduction to interview technique in:

Moser, C. and Kalton, G. (1971) *Survey Methods in Social Investigation*. Aldershot: Gower.

Sally McIntyre discusses how she made some of her decisions in her research of single mothers. The research is reported in:

McIntyre S. (1977) *Single and Pregnant*. Beckenham: Croom Helm.

McIntyre S. (1979) Some issues in the study of pregnancy carers. In: *Sociological Review* 27(4): 755–771.

The unit *Healthcare Evaluation* also looks in some depth at interview techniques.

Try writing an interview guide for an unstructured interview linked to your enquiry question. Try it out in a mock interview with a colleague. Ask your colleague to tell you at the end how he/she felt the 'interview' had gone. Note down in your learning journal the person's reactions and your thoughts on how to improve the guide.

Think if you would be more likely to give honest answers in an interview to:

- A man or a woman
- Someone from the same or a different ethnic group as yourself
- Someone who was older, the same age or younger than you.

What other characteristics of the interviewer might affect the way you responded?

How will you take these subjective responses into account if you are doing interviews for your enquiry?

Gathering data – 2

Observation

In the social sciences another way of gathering data is by observation. This involves watching subjects in a situation and recording their behaviour. It is often combined with interviewing. There are four types of observation:

- *Complete participation:* where the observer enters the setting as a member of the group and conceals his/her role as a researcher
- *Participant-as-observer:* where other members of the group are told about the researcher's dual role
- *Observer-as-participant:* where the observer spends most of the time observing the participants but also spends a small amount of time in their work role
- *Complete observer:* where the observer is a 'fly on the wall' and has no interaction with the participants.

Each type of observation has advantages and disadvantages. The main problem with complete participation is ethical — there are few situations where it can be justified. Complete participation may be acceptable if researchers might be in physical danger if they admitted what they were doing and if the research is important enough to justify the deception. On a practical level, it is very difficult to take notes as a complete observer.

Combining participant and observer roles may lead to a conflict of interests. This is particularly relevant for healthcare professionals observing in their own workplace, who may temporarily have to abandon their research role to help with a patient or client.

Complete observers don't usually have conflicts of interest, but can be inhibited by their inability to participate. Events may be happening that they don't understand, but they are unable to ask for clarification. Observations are sometimes made using video recorders. The main advantage of this is that recordings can be played back and watched carefully: but they can miss a lot out.

Field notes

Researchers carrying out observations should jot down notes of what they see, as an *aide-mémoire.* As soon as possible after leaving the field, they should write up their rough notes into full field notes.

Field notes should contain as much relevant detail as possible, including descriptions of:

- The setting — with a map, if relevant

'When I had my first baby I had prepared a birth plan and wanted to record the birth process in as much detail as possible, for my own interest. The first stage of labour was very long and I had a notebook with me in the delivery room on which I noted down the time at which various things were done. One member of staff, an agency midwife, became very alarmed when she saw me writing things down and went and complained to the midwife in charge of the ward. This incident ruined the relationship between the midwife and myself and added to the difficulties of the birth.'

'In many situations. . . data obtained from video recordings have limitations. . . a human eye subtends an angle of approximately 120 degrees but a typical 50mm camera lens covers only 25 degrees. Much that meets the eye does not, therefore, meet the lens and so even extended re-examination of a film or videotape may leave some episode defined ambiguously.'

Carr, E. K. (1991) Observational methods in rehabilitation research. *Clinical Rehabilitation* 5: 89-94.

How would you feel if you went to a party with friends and later discovered that the person you were talking to all evening was engaged in research and had been making notes of your conversation?

How would you feel if you discovered that a colleague was making secret notes on your behaviour at work for a research project?

Which type of observation would be most appropriate in the following situations?

- Observing the behaviour of illegal drug-users
- Observing the behaviour of staff in the setting where you work
- Observing the behaviour of staff in a setting where you used to work.

There is a useful introduction to observation in:

Simpson, M. and Tuson, J. (1995) *Using Observations in Small-Scale Research: A beginner's guide*. Edinburgh: Scottish Council for Research in Education.

- Who was present — a list, or more detailed descriptions of behaviour, mannerisms, etc.
- What happened
- What was said
- Non-verbal communication
- The time, date and location of the observation.

Wherever possible, the exact words of participants should be recorded. If only the approximate words are recorded, they should be placed in square brackets.

Field notes should be as objective as possible. But observers should record their own feelings about what is going on. This may reveal a subjective bias or provide an idea for later analysis.

Other methods of gathering data
Some data may come from clinical measurements, patients' records, hospital statistics or other official records. These data can be used in conjunction with data gathered in observation and interviews.

Some researchers gather material by examining the letters or diaries of subjects, or their personal accounts of their experiences. Others draw on the media. The content of all these sources can be analysed.

Your choice of method will depend on the research paradigm you are using, the kind of data you are looking for and practical and ethical considerations. You will need to be able to explain and justify your choice of method in your project.

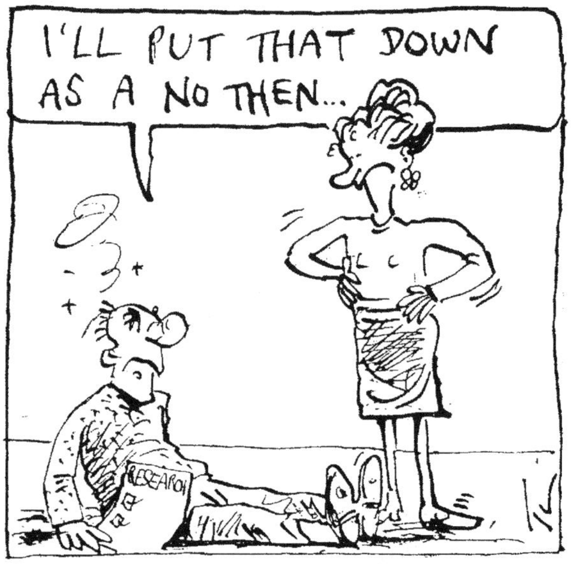

TIM SAUNDERS

Listen to what's behind the words

If someone else was going to observe you in the setting that you are in at this moment, for a research project about study methods used by healthcare professionals, what kind of details (such as setting, resources, time of day) do you think should be recorded in the researcher's field notes?

Think about the data-gathering phase of your enquiry.

- Which method or methods are you going to use to gather data?
- How would you explain and justify your decision to another person?
- What else do you need to know about these methods?
- Where are you going to get the information you need?

Here is a passage from a researcher's field notes:

10.08 S left the room. Patient A sat without moving, her knees close together, holding her handbag on her lap. She was fiddling with the strap. Her gaze was fixed on activity on a building site visible through the window.

10.15 S entered the room, and went quickly to her chair without looking at Patient A.

S: 'So sorry to have kept you'. S opened the file and began reading the notes, turning pages over rapidly, without making eye contact.

Laughter audible from staff in the adjoining office. (Did A think she was the subject of this laughter?)

A: [Are you the person who spoke to my husband?].....

Ethical issues

After the Second World War trials in Nuremberg in 1947, a code was drawn up (the Nuremberg Code) which gives 10 rules of practice for experiments on human subjects. The code underpins the World Medical Association's Declaration of Helsinki in 1964 and many subsequent codes of practice.

Informed consent

In medical research, it is necessary to obtain the informed consent of research subjects. If someone is to be given an experimental drug, or have conventional therapy withdrawn, it is right that that person should be aware of the possible consequences. Any research which involves a change in the therapy received by a patient also poses risks and informed consent is needed for this. Even if a researcher is administering only a questionnaire to patients, they may find the process time-consuming, inconvenient or stressful.

Informed consent presents two difficulties to the researcher enquiring into healthcare practice. First, if the study is a qualitative one, it is not always possible to describe the research process in detail. The researcher may know that he or she wants to interview the subject, but may not know how long the interview will take or whether it will be necessary to follow it up with other interviews. The second problem is possible conflict between the researcher's role as a researcher and as a healthcare professional. If patients agree to take part in a survey, are they agreeing because they understand your role as a researcher, or because they trust you as a healthcare professional?

This confusion of roles can also be important when observing other professionals at work. If an emergency involving patients arises during an observation, and you are qualified to help, you must do so. Other, more subtle, ethical dilemmas can also arise. What do you do if you are interviewing a patient and the patient asks you questions in your role as a healthcare professional? If you answer, you may invalidate your research. The ethical decision to take here depends on the degree of vulnerability and need of the subject.

During an observation, it is possible that a researcher will witness unprofessional or even illegal behaviour in staff. This is a difficult ethical dilemma. If patients are potentially at risk, the facts should be recorded in the research. If there is an immediate danger, the researcher should forget the research process and act to protect the patient.

War photographers are sometimes criticised for photographing atrocities and not intervening to try and prevent them.

- What do you think their duty is in these situations?
- In what way is the duty of the healthcare professional who witnesses unprofessional conduct different?

What exactly is meant by confidentiality and anonymity? You will need to decide on your own guidelines for your investigation. Is it a breach of confidentiality, for example, to make use of comments made in the staff room over a cup of tea?

'. . . you invariably find that research has an ethical or moral component; knowledge may be neutral, but the uses to which it is put may not be.'

Brooks, N. (1988) Why research? *British Journal of Occupational Therapy* 51: (11): 397-8.

Do you think that patients who benefit from the skills of healthcare professionals have any moral obligation to participate in research if it will help the development of healthcare practice?

There is an interesting discussion of this point in:

Sims, J. (1991) Nursing research: is there an obligation to participate? *Journal of Advanced Nursing* 16: 1284-89.

Confidentiality
When subjects give their consent, it is usual to guarantee confidentiality. In a large survey, this is usually easy to do.

But in a small sample of subjects, personal details in a report may make individuals readily identifiable. You should not change any information about your subjects in your report — but you can choose the information to include.

Think about the ethical implications of research while you are in the conceptual phase and stay sensitive to the issues as your work progresses.

Ethics committees
If you intend to use patients or clients as research subjects, you are likely to need permission from the ethics committee. (This is one reason to base your research on the attitudes and behaviour of other healthcare professionals.) Even if your research is not on patients, in some organisations you will still have to submit your proposal to the ethics committee. Some ethics committees meet only four times a year, so this can be a problem.

It is essential to find out what the local rules are in the organisation where you will be doing your enquiry. Talk to your tutor/counsellor, supervisor and senior managers about whether you will need to submit your proposal to the ethics committee.

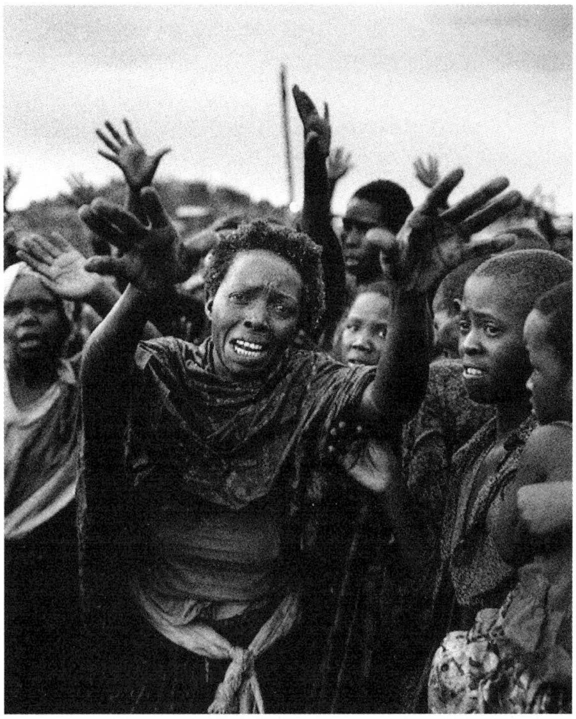

How can you observe what you are feeling - or feel what you are observing?

What rules about submission of research to an ethics committee apply in the organisation where you work? If you think you may need to get permission to go ahead with your proposed project, find out how often the committee meets and the exact conditions it sets.

'My original intention was to study the behaviour of young children visiting their mothers and newborn siblings on a maternity ward. I discovered I would need permission from the ethics committee to do this and decided instead to base my research on staff perceptions of the same behaviour.'

Might you have to modify your own research topic?

In what way could you do this?

'All of the procedures, forms, regulations and institutional review committees cannot ensure that research will be done critically unless the researcher has integrity and a commitment to a value system which considers ethical concerns and human dignity as a primary aspect of research planning.'

Fox, D. J. (1982) *Fundamentals of Research in Nursing* (4th edition). Connecticut: Appleton-Century Crofts.

Piloting and practising

Before starting to gather data, some form of piloting or other preparation may be necessary so that you can:

- Decide what data you are going to collect
- Prepare the instrument you are going to use to collect the data.

In quantitative studies, such as those involving surveys, it can be useful to conduct pilot interviews with experts or members of the target population for the survey. They help the researcher to get a 'feel' for the subject and to work out the most useful questions to ask. There is more detailed advice about piloting questionnaires for a survey on the opposite page.

In qualitative research, there are three steps you can take to prepare yourself for gathering data.

1. Practise interview technique

Interviews, particularly unstructured interviews, require skill and sensitivity on the part of the interviewer. If you are relaxed and able to ask probing questions without causing offence, you will be more effective.

Once you have prepared your questions or interview guide, practise two or three interviews with friends or colleagues and evaluate the results.

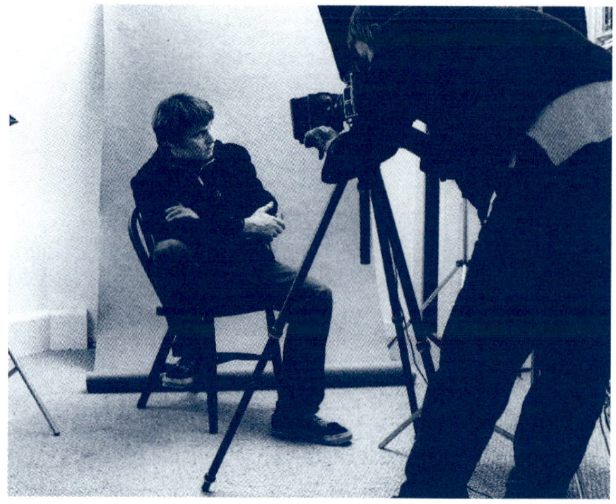

RICHARD SMITH

Getting a feel for each other: Who's in control?

2. Visit an observation site

Before conducting an observation, visit the site to introduce yourself to the participants and explain your role; for example, will you want them to ignore your presence or be ready to answer your questions as events unfold? You will also find out who the 'gatekeepers' are in the situation — the people who can give or deny you access and information. It helps to build a good relationship

A professional photographer says:

'At the beginning of a studio session, I take practice shots on instant polaroid film to check composition, lighting and exposure. After that I take the main photographs using standard film.'

Preparing to interview

1 Decide whether to tape-record or write notes during the interviews - and be clear about your reasons.

2 If you tape-record, check that the interviewee does not mind.

3 Check that the microphone is powerful enough to pick up quiet voices.

4 Check the equipment is in working order before you start.

5 Write and record on the tape or your notepad the date and time of the interview and interviewee pseudonym/number.

6 Write notes and reflections immediately afterwards.

7 Keep notes and recordings in a secure place to ensure confidentiality.

When you practise an interview, evaluate:

- How you prepared for it
- When you felt in control
- Moments when you felt awkward, confused or out of your depth
- Questions which did (and did not) provide useful answers and why this was
- Whether you phrased your questions in the most effective way
- Whether you started and finished the interview effectively
- Whether you talked too much
- If there are any other issues you should explore in the interview
- The interviewee's perception of the experience.

You could find useful information in:

Burgess, R. (1984) *In the Field: An introduction to field research*. London: Allen and Unwin.

with them. A preparatory visit may also help clarify exactly what details you need to observe and record. Is the attitude of a particular participant or the time taken for certain events significant?

3. Pilot a questionnaire

When a market research company undertakes a large-scale survey, the questionnaire is piloted extensively first, perhaps going through seven or eight versions before the final wording is decided. You do not have to go to these lengths. But you should test your questionnaire on members of the population, or individuals who are as similar to the population as possible.

The aim of the pilot is to establish whether the answers to your questions provide the sort of information you are looking for. Look at how your pilot respondents answered your questions. If you are in any doubt, ask them what they thought the question meant. After piloting, revise your questionnaire and then re-pilot it. You may have to go through this process more than once.

You may decide to re-use a questionnaire that has been designed by another researcher. If you do this, check that it was properly piloted. If you are adapting the questionnaire in any way or using it with a different population, you must re-pilot it.

It can also be helpful to pilot the way you present your questionnaire. Think about:

- The size of boxes you ask people to write in
- The size of type
- Whether people understand which parts they are not supposed to write in.

You can evaluate points such as these by interviewing your pilot respondents.

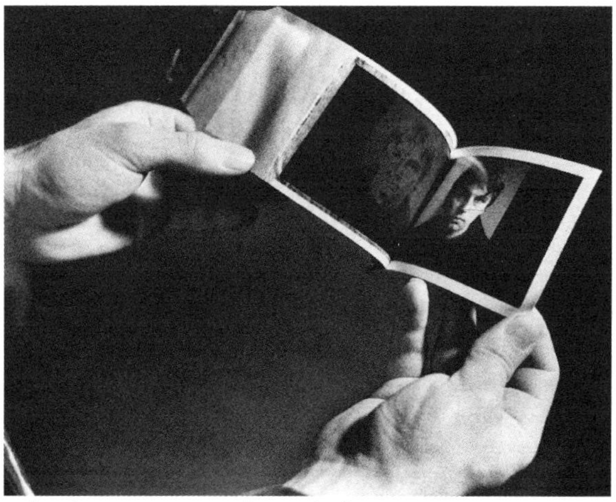

RICHARD SMITH

What have we got at the end of it?

Problematic questions

A biased or leading question influences the way people answer:

'What examples of racist behaviour have you noticed in your workplace in the past month?'

Different levels of technicality are appropriate to different audiences. Some questions may use language which is too technical:

'Has anyone in your family experienced a MCI?'

Some questions are ambiguous:

'What do you think is the best way of obtaining promotion?'

In this example, does 'best' mean 'most effective' or 'most admirable'?

There are some questions which people may be unwilling to answer:

'Have you ever failed to report a change in a patient's condition?'

There are other questions which respondents may be unable to answer, because the answer lies outside their knowledge or experience:

'Are most patients satisfied with the revised discharge procedure?'

In closed questions, where you are offering a limited range of answers, you need to be sure that the range is not too narrow:

'If you were aware that a colleague had an alcohol dependency problem that was affecting her work, would you:

1. *Report the situation to the hospital management?*
2. *Report the situation to your professional body?*
3. *Do nothing?'*

How could you improve on the wording of these questions?

Data analysis for quantitative research

In quantitative research, data are analysed using statistical methods. Some books on statistics are listed on the opposite page. These two pages give a basic outline of the subject and indicate areas which you may want to study in more detail.

Descriptive statistics

When you first obtain the results of a survey or an experiment, the data are usually in the form of a mass of numbers. In order to understand what these numbers mean, you have to sort and summarise them — hence the term descriptive statistics.

One simple form of summarising numbers is to work out an average. The three types of average (mean, median and mode) are described on pages 72 and 73.

It is also useful to know whether your results fall into a pattern — the distribution of your results. If you were to measure the height of 100 people and draw a graph to show your results, it would probably look like the graph below. All the results are placed symmetrically around the mean, with decreasing numbers of results as you go towards the upper and lower limits of the graph. It has been found that many characteristics of human beings, such as height, birth weight, resting pulse, weight and intelligence, follow a normal distribution curve like this.

Sometimes, results will be skewed to one or other end of the graph. If very few results occur below the most frequent result and the graph tails off to the right, the distribution is positively skewed. On the other hand, if the results build up slowly to the most frequent scores and then fall off quickly, the graph is negatively skewed.

It can be important to know the variability of the results, or how much they vary from the mean score. Two measures are useful. The range gives the difference between the highest and lowest score. It is also useful to know how much, on average, the results vary from the mean score. This is known as the standard deviation.

Very often, the purpose of a quantitative study is to establish whether there is a relationship between two values, such as, for example, a woman's age when she has her first baby and the length of her stay in hospital after the birth. The relationship between two values can be expressed as a figure, known as the correlation coefficient.

Bell-shaped curve of normal distribution graph - Y axis marked 'Frequency' and X axis marked 'Test score'

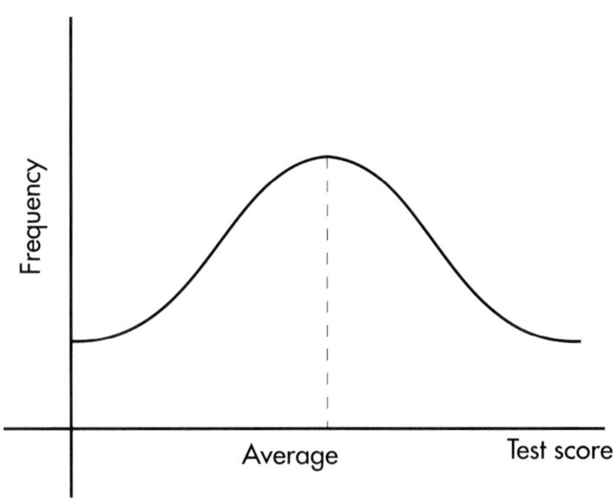

Can you think of two values, in the context of your own research project, where you would want to see whether a relationship exists?

'A variable is a quantity that can take on different values but whose value in a given situation is often unknown. It is to be contrasted with a constant quantity. The number of biological parents a person has is a constant. The number of biological offspring he or she has is a variable.'

Paulos, J.A. (1991) *Beyond Numeracy*. London: Penguin.

If the value of one variable rises as the other rises, statisticians say there is a positive correlation. If, on the other hand, the value of one variable goes down as the other rises, there is a negative correlation.

Would you expect to see a positive or a negative correlation between the following variables:

- The number of units of alcohol consumed by a subject and the length of a sequence of figures he or she is able to memorise?
- The amount of time spent studying and the mark gained in an examination?

Inferential statistics

This is the branch of statistics concerned with the estimations and predictions that can be made from data. This form of statistics allows inferences about a population to be made from observations of a sample.

Inferential statistics is based on the fact that if you take a series of different samples from a population, and arrange the mean value of each of these samples on a graph, you get a normal distribution curve - like the one on the opposite page. Some samples will have a much higher mean than the population, and some will have a much lower mean. But the majority of the samples will have a mean which is relatively close to the mean of the whole population. This distribution is known as the sampling distribution of the mean. The likely accuracy of any inferences you can make is determined by the size of the sample compared to the size of the population. It is given by a figure known as standard error of the mean.

In quantitative research, the aim is to establish whether the data support, or fail to support, a research hypothesis. As described on page 85, statisticians do this by creating a null hypothesis and testing the data against it. If the data support the null hypothesis, then the research hypothesis is not supported. The tests that are used fall into two groups: parametric tests and non-parametric tests. Parametric tests are used when at least one parameter (characteristic of the population) is known; the results are on a measured scale and it is possible to assume a normal distribution. In other situations, non-parametric tests are used. Some of these statistical tests are listed on page 73.

If you want to work out the relationships between three or more variables, multivariate statistical procedures are used.

These days, most statistical work is done on computer. This makes the process of sorting and analysing much faster and more accurate, but does not do away with the need for the researcher to understand the principles of the subject.

'probability and statistics. . . , though deep in a sense, will require nothing more than common sense and arithmetic.'

Paulos, J. A. (1988) *Innumeracy*. London: Penguin.

If you want to gain a working knowledge of statistics, the following titles will be helpful:

Polit, D.F. and Hungler, B.P. (1993) *Essentials of Nursing Research* (3rd ed). Philadelphia: J.B. Lippincott.

Polit, D.F. and Hungler, B.P. (1987) *Nursing Research: Principles and methods* (3rd ed). Philadelphia: J.B. Lippincott

Knapp, R.G. (1984) *Basic Statistics for Nurses*. (2nd ed). New Jersey: Prentice-Hall.

There is also a useful section on statistics in:

Munn, P. and Drever, E. (1995) *Using Questionnaires in Small-scale Research: A teacher's guide* (revised edition). Edinburgh: Scottish Council for Research in Education.

Use your profile to make connections between what you already know about statistics and numerical information and new things you are learning.

Talk to your tutor/counsellor about the kind of statistical analysis that will be appropriate in your project.

Check that you understand:

- How the mode, median and mean are defined
- How they are calculated
- When to use them.

Find out what computer software you have access to that will help you with statistical analysis - and how you can learn to use it.

See the units *Health Care and the Information Age* and *Healthcare Evaluation* for more about ways of analysing quantitative information.

Data analysis for qualitative research – 1

In quantitative research, most of the effort goes into collecting the data. Analysis is a relatively mechanical procedure once you understand the statistical principles involved. In qualitative research, the balance is usually the other way round. The data gathered in a qualitative study are usually in the form of recorded interviews, field notes or other written materials. The analysis is mentally demanding, time-consuming and absolutely crucial to the value and quality of the study.

The analysis of qualitative data doesn't start when the data are collected. It is a continuous process that should start as soon as the project starts. Even while data are being gathered it is possible to form ideas about analysis and interpretation — and to organise the data so that you can examine it for patterns and meaning.

Any recorded material should be transcribed and annotated with 'stage directions' which help give a fuller picture of what was going on.

Types of analysis

Codes are often used in qualitative research to group data from observations which would otherwise be impossible to analyse.

Coding is a way of capturing observations, for example of people's behaviour, so that the results of the observation can be collated and analysed.

Codes are established by the researcher before the observation takes place, and observers are trained to recognise which behaviours fit with certain codes.

The main types of analysis where coding is used are:

- *Case analysis* — this involves gathering data relevant to each particular case, whether people, services or organisations. The analysis is then written as a holistic case study.
- *Content analysis* — this involves identifying different themes and patterns in the data. Usually it is necessary to gather all the data that answer a particular question. The data are then subdivided into patterns, themes and categories.
- *Inductive analysis* — this is where patterns, themes and categories of analysis come from the data, that is, it is not being used to test a hypothesis.

Transcribing data

Decide whether you are going to write everything verbatim, including information about pauses and

'One of the greatest difficulties for evaluators engaged in qualitative analysis is that when they begin to consider causes, consequences and interdependent relationships, they fall back on quantitative analysis and begin to specify isolated variables that are mechanically linked together out of context.'

Patton, M. Q. (1987) *How to Use Qualitative Methods in Evaluation.* London: Sage Publications Ltd.

Qualitative data analysis will be particularly useful if your enquiry involves collecting data by interviewing or focus groups.

You might find it interesting to read about a recent small scale -scale qualitative study which attempted to find out what patients really want from nursing care:

Milburn, M., Baker, M.J., Gardner, P. et al. (1995) Nursing care that patients value. *British Journal of Nursing* 4(18):1094-1098.

'Imagine a large gymnasium in which thousands of toys are spread out on the floor. You are given the task of sorting them into piles according to a scheme that you are to develop. You walk around the gym looking at the toys, picking them up and examining them. There are many ways to form piles. They could be sorted according to size, colour, country of origin, date manufactured, manufacturer, material they are made from, the type of play they encourage, the age group they suit, or whether they present living things or inanimate objects.

Such an activity approaches what a qualitative researcher does to develop a coding system to organise data, though the task for the qualitative researcher is more difficult. The settings are more complex, the materials to be organised are not as easily separated into units, the setting is not void of people, nor are the classification systems as self-evident or clear-cut.'

Bogdan, R.C. and Biklen S.K. (1982) *Qualitative Research for Education: An introduction to theory and methods.* Boston: Allynn and Bacon Inc.

interruptions. These can be important if you are looking at verbal exchanges, but less important if you are interested in the participant's story and its contents. Before transcribing, listen to the tape carefully and become familiar with it.

When undertaking qualitative data analysis looking at content, keep focused on your research question and what you are trying to understand, otherwise you will find many other interesting questions also answered. One way to avoid getting sidetracked is to write down everything you know about the topic of enquiry before you start the analysis. This can help you tune into the data.

Other types of qualitative analysis include a search for key concepts which you have defined earlier.

Whatever method you choose, you should:

- Keep notes on how you went about the data analysis, so you can write this in the methodology section of your report
- Keep a record of date, interview number, speaker, line number, page number of each relevant chunk of data.

Remember that what you write now can form the foundation for the final report.

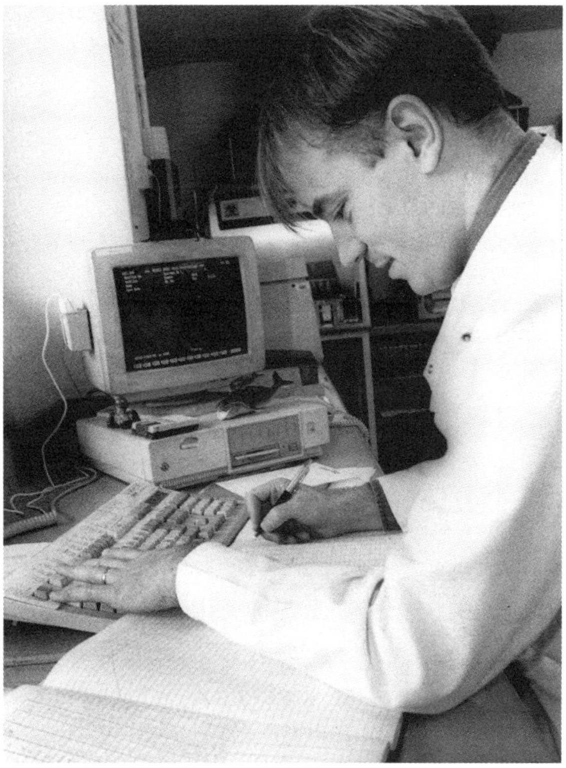

ULRIKE PRESS

Words and numbers: 'We have no time to stand and stare?' W.H. Davies, 'Leisure'. In: *Poem for the Day.* Albery, N. (ed). (1994) London: The Natural Death Centre

You can find more information about analysis of qualitative data in:

Bogdan, R.C. and Biklen S.K. (1982) *Qualitative Research for Education: An introduction to theory and methods.* Boston: Allynn and Bacon Inc.

Wolcott, H. (1994) *Transforming Qualitative Data: Description, analysis and interpretation.* Newbury Park, Ca.: Sage Publications Inc.

Chenitz, W.E. and Swanson, J.M. (1986) *From Practice to Grounded Theory.* California: Addison Wesley Publishing Company.

Gilbert, N. (ed) (1992) *Researching Social Life.* London: Sage Publications Ltd.

Holsti, O.R. (1969) *Content Analysis for the Social Sciences and Humanities.* Massachusetts: Addison-Wesley.

Corbin, J. and Strauss, L.T. (1990) *Basics of Qualitative Research.* Newbury Park, Ca.: Sage Publications Inc.

When writing about the methodology of modern science, the 16th century philosopher and scientist Francis Bacon said: 'God forbid that we should give out a dream of our imagination for a pattern of the world.'

- How can you ensure that you present things as they really are, rather than as you would like them to be?
- How can you be sure that other people are presenting you with a true 'pattern of the world' rather than a 'dream of imagination'?

Data analysis for qualitative research – 2

The data obtained from interviews or observations must be coded. The codes used will depend on the categories you are interested in. Data can be analysed for:

- Themes
- Stages in a process
- Particular words or phrases
- The setting or context in which the data were gathered
- Attitudes
- Events.

There are various ways of analysing data. In latent content analysis, you examine each part in the context of the whole and look for underlying meanings. In manifest content analysis, you look for key words and phrases, which can then be counted and displayed using descriptive statistics. Latent content analysis is used more frequently in qualitative research because, although it may be subjective, it has a higher validity.

The categories used to sort the data may not be clear when you start the analysis. Qualitative researchers often start with a few broad categories. As they become more familiar with the material, they make finer and finer distinctions. This may mean that you have to work through the data several times. Once you are satisfied with the categories you have identified, you can go on to interpret the data. In practice, you will almost certainly develop ideas about interpretation while you are still coding.

Sometimes you start off with a lot of coded data, perhaps coded under 20 or more categories. Grouping data under the same relevant category helps you to recognise the relationship between each chunk of data. It also helps you write a description of the category. In this process, you may transfer some material to another category, or decide it is not relevant. You may also find that some categories can be combined — it is a process of reducing and refining them. You then identify relationships and start to describe a theme which represents the different categories of data. The diagram on the opposite page represents this relationship between theme, categories and data.

If you want to present a theme in your report, you should be able to identify and locate a chunk of data which fits best and can be traced back to its origins.

The following is a possible layout for a transcribed interview. Type what is said in the left hand column. Add other information about tone of voice, actions, and so on, in a second column and add coding information in a third column.

What is said	Tone of voice, actions	Coding information
A: I don't know what can have happened to her. She said she would be here.		
M: It's only just gone half past.	Placatory	
A: I told her not to be late...she knows you were both coming along today.	Getting angry	
M: It's not important, really. Perhaps she wasn't...		
A: She's always doing this...letting me down.	Starting to cry	
M: Come on, it really doesn't matter. We can get started without her.	Opens briefcase	

The English word 'measure' comes from the same root as the Sanskrit word 'maya', meaning 'illusion'. Eastern philosophy regards the immeasurable as the primary reality — as when we say 'I've got the measure of her'.

How far do you think qualitative analysis can reflect the truth?

Bohm, D. (1980) *Wholeness and the Implicate Order*. London: Ark.

Practical techniques

The aim of analysis is to describe each section of the data and identify it in such a way that everything relating to a particular category can be retrieved and compared.

The traditional way to do this is to use McBee cards. These are filing cards with a series of punched holes along the top edge. Each hole represents a different category. If a card relates to a category, the hole is left intact. When a metal rod is pushed through a hole, all the cards relevant to that category are picked up.

Nowadays, the task can be performed much more easily and efficiently by using a computer database. Whatever method you use to analyse your data, it is essential to keep at least one copy of the original material intact.

Grounded theory

This is a highly structured and thorough method of analysing qualitative data. Data are placed into categories in a similar way to other types of qualitative analysis, but great importance is placed on written memos which explore and record every step of the analytical process. The researcher continually looks across all the data to check different examples of a category. Sometimes categories are sub-divided, and sometimes several categories are combined. When no new characteristics emerge for a category, it is said to be 'saturated'. Abstract definitions of categories are prepared and these are used to build theories and to compare the findings with existing theories about the subject.

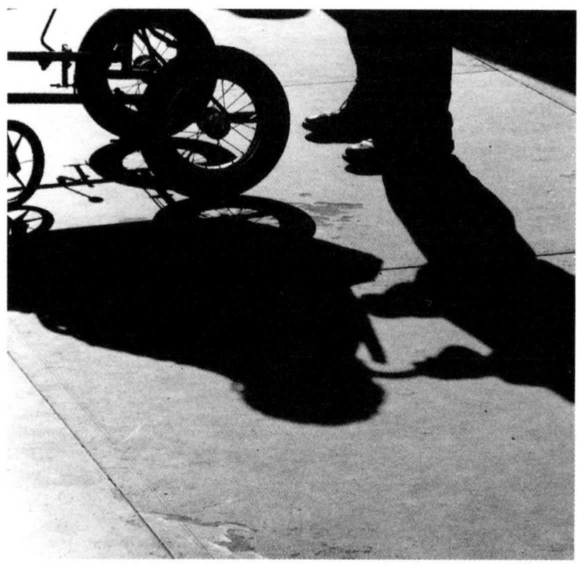

DAVID GIBSON

Are things what they seem?

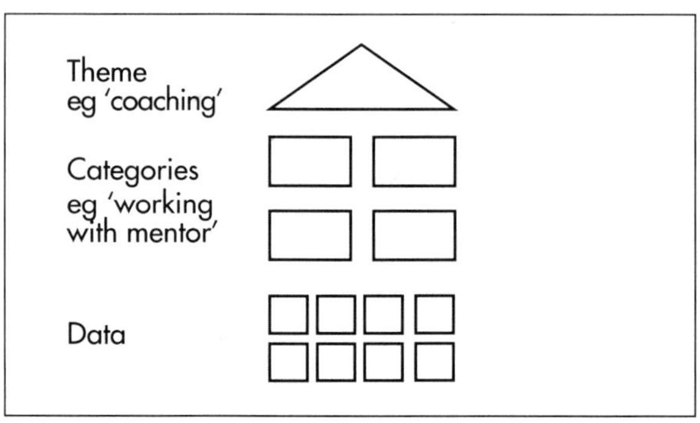

Two useful books about using computers to analyse qualitative data are:

Teck, R. (1990) *Qualitative Research: Analysis types and software tools*. London: Falmer Press.

Fielding, N. and Lee, R. (1990) *Using Computers in Qualitative Research*. London: Sage Publications.

If you do not know the ways in which information can be sorted using a computer database, talk to someone who does or see the unit entitled *Health Care and the Information Age*.

Think about the issues you are exploring in your enquiry.

- What types of categories might it be useful to start with when you are coding the data?
- How could you use the possibilities offered by a computer database to organise and retrieve data?

Results, interpretation, conclusions and recommendations

After the data are analysed, researchers should be ready to:

- Summarise the results
- Offer an interpretation of what they mean
- Draw conclusions from the study
- Make recommendations based upon these conclusions.

Quantitative research

When you present your results, start with a general outline of your findings. It will probably be useful to illustrate this with descriptive statistics, such as averages (see pages 72-73) or standard deviations (see page 100). You can then go on to use inferential statistics to discuss the importance of your results (see page 101). It is usual to name the statistical tests used and to give the level of statistical significance. Readers will need this kind of information to check the reasoning and decide whether they agree with your conclusions.

Remember, you cannot say that your hypothesis is 'proved' or 'disproved' by your results. All you can say is that it is 'supported' or 'not supported'. Statistical analysis is concerned with probabilities and cannot lead to certainty.

If your results do show a correlation between the variables in your hypothesis, be careful about identifying cause and effect. Your recommendations can suggest further work that could be done to investigate this relationship.

A mistake that many people make is to allow their conclusions and recommendations to go far beyond their data. This can happen in situations where the researcher has a very strong intuitive idea of what is happening in a situation and of what should be done as a result.

If the findings do not support the hypothesis in the way you expected, it is essential to recognise this fact. It may be that your hypothesis was wrong. This is a state of affairs that many researchers are reluctant to admit. It could also be that there was something wrong with the way you designed or carried out your study. If you can see limitations of this kind, you will be doing others a service if you discuss them.

In the end, it is not whether your data supported or failed to support the hypothesis that is important, but the rigour with which you interpret data. A flawed study in which the flaws are examined is much more valuable than a flawed study in which the shortcomings are glossed over.

An example of how results should be described:

The mean reaction time for subjects under the control condition was 0.35 seconds, while under the eight pint condition it was 0.54 seconds. This difference was tested using the repeated measures t-test and found to be significant, with df = 18, significance level = 0.05, t = 5.12.

In a criminal trial, guilt has to be proved 'beyond all reasonable doubt'.

How does this compare with the relationship between the results of a research study and the recommendations that can be made?

In October 1995, preliminary research findings were released about possible side-effects of some low dosage contraceptive pills. The UK government reacted immediately by recommending that women using these pills consult their doctors. The research establishment considered this recommendation to be unwarranted.

Very occasionally, the results of a research study are so startling that it is possible to make immediate recommendations for changes in practice. More usually, the results are less clear-cut and the recommendations concern further research that should be done.

What kind of recommendations do you think you will be able to make from your enquiry?

Qualitative research

When reporting a qualitative study, it is important to capture and convey a sense of the particular reality your research was looking at. Qualitative researchers, as well as quantitative researchers, should try to 'stay close to the data' in the sense of not making assertions that are not supported by the study. Qualitative research is not usually generalisable to other situations, so you should avoid the temptation of suggesting that your findings have wider implications than in fact they have.

One well known danger for qualitative researchers is 'going native'. This happens when a researcher becomes completely won over by the perceptions and attitudes of the participants and loses all sense of objectivity.

One way to guard against rash interpretations of results is to discuss them with friends and colleagues. You may be surprised at the different explanations that they can offer for the phenomena you observed.

At the end of a qualitative study, you are unlikely to be able to offer definite recommendations for changes in practice. But you may be able to share:

- Insights which other healthcare professionals will find helpful in their practice
- The development of a theory
- An understanding of how an existing theory applies in a particular context
- Hypotheses which could be tested out in further research - perhaps of a quantitative nature.

'I am appalled by the frequent publication of papers that describe most minutely what experiments were done, and how, but with no hint of why or what they mean. Cast thy data upon the waters, the authors seem to think, and they will come back interpreted.

Woodford, P. F. (1967) Sounder thinking through clearer writing. *Science* 156 (3776): 743-45.

Here are some of the ways in which one researcher thought her research findings (in which she identified three 'caring career' patterns for informal carers of people with dementia) could be applied:

- Helping doctors to realise the significance on the carers of a formal diagnosis
- Helping doctors and other medical staff to appreciate how the information they provide on caring implications may affect the experience of carers
- Helping policy-makers and managers to understand how the needs of informal carers for day care and support change over time.

Taraborrelli, P. (1992) Becoming a carer. In: Gilbert, N. (ed) *Researching Social Life*. London: Sage Publications Ltd.

'Researchers weaned on quantitative methods may succumb to overwhelming urges to reduce their qualitative data to numerical categories or neat variables, seeking to achieve respectability for their results at the cost of more penetrating analyses (or interpretations) that might raise questions rather than put them ever to rest.'

Wolcott, H. (1994) *Transforming Qualitative Data: Description, analysis and interpretation*. Newbury Park, Ca.: Sage Publications Inc.

'The TV scientist who mutters sadly, "The experiment is a failure; we have failed to achieve what we had hoped for," is suffering mainly from a bad scriptwriter. The experiment is never a failure solely because it fails to achieve predicted results. An experiment is a failure only when it also fails adequately to test the hypothesis in question, when the data it produces don't prove anything one way or the other.'

Pirsig, R. M. (1975) *Zen and the Art of Motorcycle Maintenance*. New York: Bantam.

Limitations

Very few research projects can be described as perfect. Some compromises may have to be made before you even start. For example, you might want to do a survey of the emotional needs of people with AIDS but find that it is impossible to obtain a random sample. Instead, you have to rely on a network of contacts to identify individuals who are willing to participate in your research. Findings from this sample may be useful, but they will not have the same meaning as they would if the sample were random. In this situation, it might be appropriate to take another approach, such as undertaking a phenomenological study.

In other situations, you may not have the resources to use as large a sample as you might want. This will affect the statistical significance of the results.

If your research is based on observation, you may not be allowed to enter certain areas or to be present at particular times. Participants may insist that you make definite appointments for your visits and make sure that anything they don't want you to see happens at times when you are not present. Other problems may happen while you are doing your research. For example, participants may explicitly withdraw their support - or simply fail to return your questionnaires.

You may find that:

- You have unknowingly stepped into a situation where strong political forces affect the way participants respond to questions. For example, if you are interviewing staff about their level of job satisfaction, you may get untypical results if the unit they work in is threatened with imminent closure.
- The people you chose to interview are not as knowledgeable about a subject as you first imagined, or that they have particular characteristics or circumstances which make them untypical
- It is very difficult to keep your personal admiration or dislike of an individual separate from your interpretation of the data with which you are being provided. Alternatively, a participant may have a strong personal reaction to you as an individual
- A particular source of data is not as useful as you thought it was going to be. For example, you might decide to do a content analysis of health promotion booklets produced by a number of different health authorities and

Talk to other healthcare professionals who have undertaken research. Share your experiences of problems. You might like to do this on the Internet, where you will be able to communicate with people in similar situations to yourself all over the world.

'Objectivity, in short, has the logical status of a myth: it builds up one sense of reality rather than others. It is a myth whose attainment and maintenance demands of its subjects a rigorous and continued asceticism. . .'

Novak, M. (1970) *The Experience of Nothingness.* New York: Harper and Row.

It is impossible to be completely objective. But it is possible to be aware of the preconceptions and beliefs which may affect your conclusions and recommendations. Use your learning journal to help you keep track.

The unit *Influences in Health Care: Media perspectives* has interesting insights how information is presented.

'I underestimated the suspicion that people might have about answering my questionnaire. I should have taken more care to reassure them about confidentiality. If I'd done that, I might have had more co-operation.'

'I didn't realise it, but I was the third healthcare professional to ask to interview a certain key individual in the past month. No wonder she turned me down.'

'I was analysing my interview transcripts on cut up pieces of paper. The only copy of the original was in my car when it was stolen.'

'It was only on my last observation that I realised I should have been noting the time it took someone to perform a particular activity on different occasions. This information was absolutely critical to my understanding of the situation - but I didn't realise it until too late.'

'There was a scare in the newspapers about unauthorised people walking around the wards of a hospital. The management was feeling very sensitive and, in the middle of my observations, refused me permission to visit without a prior appointment.'

then discover that most of the booklets had been based on the same source material.

As a novice, you may also make practical errors, such as underestimating the time it will take you to analyse results.

All the difficulties described on the opposite page can interfere with the validity of a study. It is essential that you recognise these problems and discuss their implications, even if you feel a little foolish about admitting some of your 'mistakes'.

Your assessor will not be expecting perfection and will be much more interested in seeing how you negotiated obstacles and knowing that you understand the limitations of your study. When you are writing up your report, you should mention limitations when describing your methods and review them in more detail when discussing your results. The limitations of your study may provide useful material for the recommendations you make for further enquiry.

On a personal level, it can be frustrating if the reality of your enquiry does not meet up with expectations. It may seem that you have put in a tremendous amount of effort to achieve much less than you hoped.

But enquiry often advances in this slow, painstaking way. And, paradoxically, the more difficulties you have encountered in your study, the more you are likely to have learned from the experience. Not only will you be in a better position to understand and criticise the research of others, but you will also be able to develop your techniques if you do further research in the future.

Look back at the discussion of internal and external validity on pages 54 and 55.

What challenges to the validity of your study did you encounter?

'If you will tell me why the fen appears impassable, I then

will tell you why I think that I

can get across it if I try.'

Marianne Moore, 'I may, I might, I must.' In: Albery, N. (ed). (1994) *Poem for the Day*. London: The Natural Death Centre.

It is important not to lose sight of your original purpose and aims. These can form criteria to help you evaluate what you are learning and how you are learning.

In your reflective diary, list:

- Three things you are proud of achieving in your research
- Three insights you have gained as a result of doing your research
- Three things you would do differently if you were to start again now.

Conclusion

This Section has been right through the process of planning and carrying out an enquiry-based project. If you have been doing the project at the same time as working through the Section, you should by now have:

- Collected your data
- Analysed it
- Thought about what conclusions and recommendations you can make.

The value of going through this process does not lie only in the importance of your findings. It may well be that you have gained useful insights which you will be able to incorporate into your own practice. You will also now have a stronger understanding of what enquiry can, and cannot, achieve, and also of the implications of the decisions taken at every stage.

Section 5 describes how to communicate findings from your enquiry to other people.

Not to say what everyone else was saying
not to believe what everyone else believed
not to do what everybody did,
then to refute what everyone else was saying
then to disprove what everyone else believed
then to deprecate what everybody did,
Was his way to come by understanding
how everyone else was saying the same as he was saying
believing what he believed
and did what he was doing.

Clere Parsons, 'Different'. In: Albery, N. (ed.) (1994) *Poem for the Day*. London: The Natural Death Centre.

References

Leedy, P. (1989). The review of related literature. In: Leedy, P. *Practical Research: Planning and design.* (4th edition) New York: Macmillan.

Taraborrelli, P. (1992) Becoming a carer. In: Gilbert, N. (ed). *Researching Social Life.* London: Sage Publications Ltd.

'I never travel without my diary. One should always have something sensational to read on the train.' — Oscar Wilde

Use your learning journal or reflective diary or a small notebook to record sensations and the ways you come to understanding. Sometimes they come unexpectedly.

Introduction

Writing a report (or assessment) comes last, when all the work of data collection and analysis has been done. For some people, this is the best bit: writing clarifies their interpretation of results, helps them to see what the enquiry has achieved and allows their findings to be made known to a wider audience.

Other people find the idea of writing up their report quite intimidating. They may not be confident writers, they find the material difficult to handle in writing — even through they can talk about it — and they are anxious about the moment when their work joins the 'literature' and can be compared with the efforts of other researchers and enquirers.

There are clear guidelines on the way reports can be presented, and these are explained in this Section. These guidelines on the structure, layout and language of reports are important because they help researchers to present results consistently. They can also be a useful reference point when the writing gets hard. The Section also has suggestions which may be helpful if you are not used to producing a written piece of work of any length.

At the end of the Section other ways of presenting your findings to different audiences are discussed. If you have gained insights from your study, you may wish to share them with other members of your profession in these ways.

One tutor/counsellor advises students like this:

'Writing the report should be a continuous activity, with several sections being written at the same time. Write the literature review section quite early on in the project, rather than leaving it to the end.'

Writing up your work as you go along makes the whole process seem much more possible. It also helps to create new ideas.

Don't forget that your journal or diary may be a rich source of material for your final report.

'Sometimes just the act of writing down the problems straightens out your head as to what they really are.'

Pirsig, R. M. (1975) *Zen and the Art of Motorcycle Maintenance*. New York: Bantam.

While you are writing, ask yourself questions such as these:

- What exactly do I want to say?
- Why do I want to say it?
- How can I say it most effectively?
- To whom am I saying it?

These books and articles have helpful advice on writing:

Marshall, L. and Rowland, F. (1983) *A Guide to Learning Independently*. Milton Keynes: Open University Press.

Woodford, P. (1967) Sounder thinking through clearer writing. *Science* 156 (3776): 743-45.

Strunk, W. and White, E. B. (1979) *The Elements of Style* (3rd edition). New York: Macmillan.

Elbow, P. (1973) *Writing Without Teachers*. Oxford: Oxford University Press.

How to present a research report

There is an established format for research reports. Quantitative studies should be reported using this format. Qualitative studies may depart from some aspects of it. For example, in ethnographic studies, literature, data and discussion are sometimes combined in several thematic sections.

Title

The title is not the same as the problem addressed by the enquiry, although it will contain similar information. It should show the reader:

- What kind of study it is
- The issues it looks at
- The population studied.

The following is an example of a title which tells readers what they can expect to find in the report: 'Doctors and nurses: a content analysis of gender stereotyping in television soap operas with a medical setting'.

Abstract

This contains a brief summary of the aims, methods, main results and conclusions of the study. It should not be more than one or one-and-a-half pages long. The aim is to give readers enough information to decide whether the report is relevant to their interests.

Introduction/background

This explains the importance of the study and why it was done. It is helpful to give a brief overview of each section.

Literature review

This section is discussed in detail on pages 116-117.

Methods

The research method and the methods used to collect and analyse data are described in this section, as are any instruments used, such as a questionnaire or measurement scale (these documents should be included in the appendices). The methods section should give readers all the relevant details for their understanding of the study, such as the size of the sample or the timing and place of observations.

Results

This section summarises the analysis of the data, but does not offer interpretations. Graphs and tables are often included in this section.

A detective novel falls into three parts. In the first part, the crime is committed. In the second part, the investigation takes place. In the third part the crime is solved. Many other kinds of writing have this 'three act structure'.

Can you see how it is reflected in the way a research report is organised?

Think about the order in which you read other people's research reports.

- What kind of information do you need at each stage?
- What makes you decide whether to read the full report?

- Title
- Abstract
- Acknowledgements (where necessary)
- Table of contents
- Table of illustrations and diagrams (where appropriate)
- Introduction/background
- Literature review
- Methods
- Results
- Discussion
- Conclusions and recommendations
- References/bibliography
- Appendices.

Extensive pieces of 'raw' data, such as sections of interview transcripts, should be placed in the appendices and referred to in this section.

Discussion

This is where researchers interpret their results and discuss any limitations of the study. Short samples of data are used to support the conclusions.

Conclusions and recommendations

The main body of the report is ended by summarising your conclusions and discussing any implications of the study for theory, practice or further research.

Most people don't read a research report from cover to cover. They dip in and out, looking at items in the appendices and cross-referring from the methods to the results. It is important to give readers signposts which help them to find the parts they want to read next. The traditional way to do this is number the paragraphs and sub-paragraphs within each section. These numbers should be placed in a wide, left-hand margin, with sub-headings to mark a new topic or point in the argument.

The language of research reports

Avoid colloquialism and emotive language. Use technical terms where they are needed, but do not add 'jargon' where it is unnecessary. Try to express the meaning as clearly and concisely as possible. In reports of quantitative studies, it is usual to avoid the first person singular. In qualitative research, where the actions and reactions of the researcher are often central to the study, it is often necessary to use the first person.

Using graphs and tables

Use computer software if you can to produce graphs and tables. Many word-processing packages include this facility.

Keep graphs and tables simple and straightforward. Do not be seduced by the ease with which you can produce 3-D effects or mullet-coloured pie charts. Readers are interested in what the data show, not in fancy ways of presenting it. Take care not to mislead readers - for example, by using different types of scale on two graphs you want them to compare. Graphs, tables and diagrams should be numbered and listed in their own table of contents.

Read a selection of published research reports and notice the language they use.

- What kinds of verbs do they use - state, indicate, demonstrate etc.?
- Are the sentences passive or active?
- Is the report written in the first person (I interviewed) or the third person (the researcher interviewed)?
- Does the use of language clarify or mystify?

Information about writing up findings is in:

Spradley, J. (1980) *Participant Observation.* London: Holt Rinehart & Winston.

'Then you should say what you mean,' the March Hare went on.

'I do,' Alice hastily replied; 'at least – at least I mean what I say – that's the same thing, you know.'

Carroll, L. (1970) *The Annotated Alice.* London: Penguin.

'Excellence in statistical graphics consists of complex ideas communicated with clarity, precision and efficiency. Graphical displays should:

- Show the data
- Induce the viewer to think about the substance rather than about methodology, graphic design, the technology of graphic production, or something else
- Avoid distorting what the data have to say
- Present many numbers in a small space
- Make large data sets coherent
- Encourage the eye at several levels of detail — from a broad overview to the fine structure
- Serve a reasonably clear purpose: description, exploration, tabulation, or decoration
- Be closely integrated with the statistical and verbal descriptions of a data set.'

Tufte, E. R. (1992) *The Visual Display of Quantitative Information.* Connecticut: Graphics Press.

Managing the writing process

Many people find that they need extended periods of uninterrupted time when they come to write up their enquiry. Others can give their full concentration for only an hour or two at a stretch. Be conscious of your own work patterns and their implications for your writing schedule and other responsibilities.

Although the writing task may appear daunting, it can be broken down into stages.

Getting ready

Before you start, look through all the data again and read any notes you made while planning your research and gathering and analysing data. This can also be a moment when it is especially valuable to read your reflective journal. Make the physical preparations to ensure your working environment is how you want it.

Do a rough plan

Start by doing a rough plan of what you are going to write about. You already have an overall structure of the report (see pages 112-113). Think about the points you want to cover within each section. You may find it helpful to draw diagrams which clarify the relationship between different ideas you want to include. Some people like to use an outlining feature on a word processor; others prefer pencil and paper. Use whatever technique works for you.

First draft

For many people, this is the most alarming moment. It is important not to worry unduly about the first draft. It is much better to get something down on paper, even if it's not exactly what you want to say. Finish whole sections of your report in first draft before you take them to the next stage.

There is no need to write your report in the order in which you will present it. Some sections that appear near the beginning, such as the introduction and abstract, should be written last. Some people find it best to start with the methods section, because this is the material they are most familiar with and confident about describing.

When you have finished the first draft of a section, check it over. Don't worry about details of spelling or grammar at this stage — it is more important to consider whether you

---

Write a checklist of what you need to prepare your report. For example, you might need:

- Access to a computer
- A good dictionary
- An imminent deadline - if you don't have plenty of time to write
- Complete silence in which to work
- Long periods when you are able to work without interruption
- Extra child care, or increased co-operation from other members of the family

How will you get what you need? Write an action plan.

If you know what you want to say, but are not sure about the order it should go in, you could write your points on small self-adhesive notes, then arrange and re-arrange them on a page until you are satisfied you have found a logical structure.

Or you could try drawing a very large mind map on an A1 pad to represent your report. It can be helpful to see the whole of the contents on a single sheet of paper.

'I might have to set anything from a day to a week aside for "cranking up". I might find that I have two or three clear days that I can give over to making a start on writing, to generate a bit of impetus that may then be carried on over the next two to three weeks. This is an average time for getting to grips with a writing project, and in general, I find that I have to devote all my attention to it during that period if I am to master it. I am very unsociable and rather ill-tempered during this time. Some of us may actually have to appear to undergo profound personality changes in order to do the work. Unlike Dr Jekyll, however, we have no magic potions.'

Woods, P. (1985) Creativity and technique in writing up qualitative research. In: Burgess, R.G. (ed.) *Issues in Educational Research: Qualitative methods*. Lewes: Falmer Press.

have missed out anything important and whether your argument makes sense. Have you managed to put down what's in your mind?

Second draft

Having read over your first draft, you might find you want to rewrite it completely. Or it might be near enough to what you want to say for you to do some editing. It is often best to work through the second draft of an entire section before starting to edit and correct your work. If you try to perfect every paragraph as you write it, you may make discouragingly slow progress. It is also important to see the individual parts in the context of the whole.

Edit and check

When you have finished your second draft, edit for grammar and style. Put it through a spell-check if you are using a word processor, then check it for internal consistency. It is very easy to spell names in different ways at different points, or to capitalise in different ways. Make sure that all the cross-references are up-to-date and that the numbering system is still accurate. It is a good idea to make a few general 'sweeps' through your work, checking a particular feature or type of detail each time.

Leave a day or so between finishing your report and the date you have scheduled for the printing and binding of your final version. Before you produce a final version, re-read it from cover to cover. Once you have been away from it for a couple of days, you may find last-minute improvements you can make.

It is good to have someone else to read and comment on your work as you are writing it. Don't leave it until the end when it is too late.

Your tutor/counsellor may be prepared to discuss individual sections of your report with you as you complete them. Find out what help he or she is able to give you as you write the report.

'The writer wandered to the water cooler, washed his hands, looked up the weather report, made some unnecessary phone calls, looked at his tongue in the mirror for symptoms of fatal disease and, when he had at last exhausted methods of killing time, went to his typewriter.'

Baker, R. (1972) At lunch. In: Frank, J. *You*. New York: Harcourt, Brace & Jovanovich.

Look back at the guidelines for critiquing reports on page 69.

How does your own report stand up?

A good proof reader will pick up 98 per cent of the mistakes each time they go through a typescript.

Writer's block is something that troubles many people - and professional writers have devised many ways to get around it. None of them is foolproof. But if you get blocked you might try one of these ideas.

'I write anything - it doesn't matter if it is complete nonsense - just to break the tension of having a blank page in front of me.'

'I go out for a walk.'

'I find someone who is prepared to listen while I explain what it is I am trying to write.'

'I promise myself a treat in half an hour if I get started. At the end of half an hour, I'm usually so involved that I postpone the treat.'

If you have a psychological trick which works for you, you might like to share it with other students.

How to present a literature review

These two pages discuss how you should present the literature review — and any other references to published or unpublished material — in your report. The key point to remember is that you should be presenting a discussion of what has been written about the subject, not an undigested summary.

Plan the literature review with the same care you use on any other part of your report. The review should have a clear structure, which may be based around different aspects of the problem addressed in your enquiry. If you have used network theory to organise your review, you will be aware of the relationship between different texts. Show that you are aware which are the classic or seminal works on a subject and how ideas have been developed and refined over time.

This advice to students from a colleague was quoted in an article by Paul Leedy (1989):

- Present your own discussion
- Paraphrase (précis, résumé, a synopsis, an epitome)
- Use short, direct quotations if necessary
- Long quotations are a last resort. Use them only for a very good reason.

References

References tell readers where they can find material referred to in the text. They are also a way of acknowledging the influence of other writers and researchers on your work. The Harvard system is one accepted way to present references. It is used in this book

- Names and dates are given in the body text and the full reference is listed at the end of the work.
- If the author has more than one publication in the same year, and both of these are used as a reference, they may distinguished in the text as, for example, Lancaster (1985a) and Lancaster (1985b).
- All direct quotations are in quotation marks. Put short quotations in the text and long quotations in separate, indented paragraphs.

Plagiarism

It is essential to give references for any quotations or information from other people's work, both in the literature review and anywhere else in your report. If you try to pass other people's ideas off as your own, you are guilty of plagiarism, which your assessors will view as a serious offence. One way of avoiding plagiarism is to read the relevant passage and then set it aside before writing down in your own words what you found significant.

> 'Avoid regurgitating the structure of your sources in your work. I already know what Elster has to say about functionalism (and the order in which he says it), I want to know what you think.'
>
> *Advice from Colin Mills to sociology students at the University of Surrey, Department of Sociology, 1991.*

> 'Where there is much desire to learn, there of necessity will be much arguing, much writing, many opinions; for opinion in good men is but knowledge in the making.'
>
> Milton, J. In: Marshall, L. and Rowland, F. (1983) *A Guide to Learning Independently.* Milton Keynes: Open University Press.

> If you are quoting from interview transcripts, you have an ethical obligation not to alter the wording, even if this would make your point more clearly, nor to quote out of context. It is acceptable to leave out words, as long as you make it clear to your reader that you have done so.

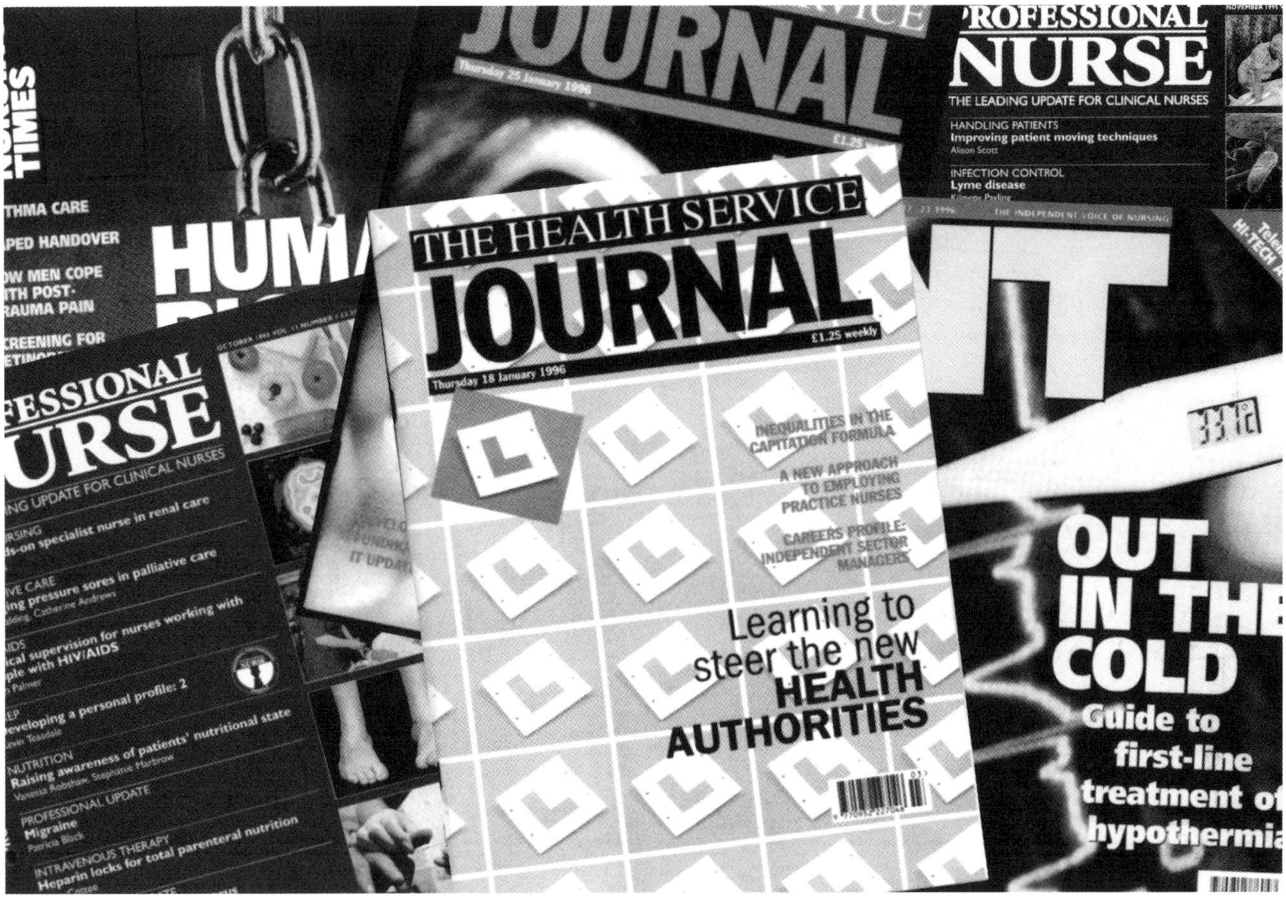

STEVE SULLIVAN

Journals provide an up-to-date resource library

How to give a reference to a book

List references alphabetically under the author's name. Give the following details:

- Author's name, followed by initials
- Year of publication, in brackets. Where there is more than one edition, the year should refer to the edition from which the reference was taken
- Title of work, underlined or in italics
- Edition of work, if more than one. Reprints need not be mentioned
- Volume number, if there is more than one volume
- Place of publication or town of origin
- Publisher's name.

How to give a reference to a journal article

Give the following information:

- Author's name, followed by initials
- Year of publication, in brackets
- Title of the article.
- Title of the journal, in full, underlined or in italics or bold
- Volume number. The date is not always necessary but can help the reader to locate a particular issue
- Issue number. This is not essential if the page numbers run on throughout the year, but again it can help the reader
- The number of the first and last pages on which the article appeared.

It is customary to use capital letters for the author's surname, and for the first letter of the first word of the title.

When the author and the publisher are the same, as sometimes happens when reports are published by organisations, the name must be repeated.

Where there is more than one author, these should be given in the text.

Committee reports are listed, both in the text and in the references, under the name of the body which was responsible for publication, not the name of the chairman of the committee.

Where do you go from here?

Once you have finished your report and handed it in, you may feel that that is the end of the enquiry-based project. But there are other ways in which you could communicate your findings to other healthcare professionals.

Some reports can provide the basis of an article. Your own work may not be on the scale of the research that is reported in some of the major journals, but it could still find a place. Once you have identified a suitable journal, look carefully at the style of the articles it contains. You will have to rewrite your report using a similar approach.

Cormack (1986) suggests this possible structure for a research article:

- Aims and objectives 15%
- Literature review 10%
- Data collection methods 10%
- Data analysis 10%
- Findings 30%
- Conclusions/recommendations for future research 25%

If you don't feel that your report could be the basis of an article, there may be other ways of communicating it more widely. If the study has implications for practice, it might be of interest to an in-house staff journal. Health authorities also like to include news of relevant developments in their annual reports, especially if they are in line with current policy initiatives. A small paragraph here could bring your study to the attention of other people who could benefit from it.

Your study may be relevant to a clinical or research conference. Some of the most interesting papers presented at conferences are on small undergraduate studies. Your tutor/counsellor should be able to advise you on preparing your work for an audience of this kind.

Another, less public, alternative is to communicate your findings in the form of a seminar or a presentation, either to other students or to a more general audience of health-care professionals.

Some studies produce ideas or information which can be made into posters. You could contact other professionals on the Internet who might be interested in reading about your research. Or you could think about putting a summary of your findings on the World Wide Web.

Look at the journals produced for healthcare professionals - academic and non-academic titles.

- Would your research be of any interest to the readers of these journals?
- If so, in what style should it be written?
- Are the percentages quoted above reflected in the journals you look at?

'In order for nursing to develop as a research-based profession, research into nursing must be undertaken and the results made widely available. One means of disseminating research-based nursing knowledge is by publishing articles in journals such as *Nurse Education Today*.'

Cormack, D.F.S. Writing a research article. *Nurse Education Today* 6: 64-68.

'We have finished the job. What shall we do with the tools?'

Telegram from the Emperor Haille Selassie of Abyssinia to Winston Churchill in 1941.

Think about what you know about the research done by other professionals who are doing research similar to your own.

- Are there any mechanisms for finding out more about the work of other individuals in your local area?
- If not, could you set them up?

The needs of different audiences

When adapting your report for another format, you need to think about the interests and concerns of your new audience. You may have to explain or simplify some technical aspects of your work, or place it in a different context.

Strauss and Corbin (1990) suggest some possible interests of different types of readers:

Academic colleagues are likely to be interested in papers whose major focus is:
- Theoretical
- Substantive
- Argumentative
- Methodological.

Practitioners are likely to be interested in:
- Theoretical frameworks for understanding clients better
- Practical suggestions for better procedures
- Reforms of existing practices
- Broad policy suggestions.

Lay readers may be more interested in:
- Reforms of current practices or policies
- Guidelines for how to manage better or get better service from practitioners or institutions
- Assurances that others share their own experience - as in living through a divorce or adopting a child.

Even if you decide not to communicate the results of your study to a wider audience, it is very likely that, after completing this unit, your own awareness and appreciation of research has been greatly increased. This will in itself contribute to the development and implementation of enquiry into healthcare practice.

Programme for a study day entitled: 'The Good Sex Guide — After cancer?' based on a research study

9.00–9.15	Registration	
9.15–9.30	Alison Wetherall–Chairperson *Oncology Services Manager*	Opening Remarks
9.30–10.30	Dr Jane Apperley *Consultant Haematologist* *Hammersmith Hospital*	Overview of causes of infertility
10.30–11.00	Coffee	
11.00–11.40	Margaret Moody *Senior Registrar in Clinical Oncology, Addenbrooke's*	Breast and gynaecological cancer – effects on sexual health
11.40–12.00	Mr Bullock *Consultant Urologist* *Addenbrooke's*	A surgeon's approach to impotency
12.00–12.10	Discussion	
12.10–12.30	Amanda Baxter *Clinical Nurse Specialist* *Pelvic Cancer*	Looking at practical approaches to sexuality issues
12.30–1.40	Lunch	
1.40–2.00	Carol Lack *Research Student* Dr Richard Osborne *Consultant in Medical Oncology*	Preliminary results of a study of the psychosocial impact of ovarian cancer diagnosis
2.00–2.30	Dr Helen Hutchinson *Senior Clinical Medical Officer, Family Planning*	Psycho-sexual counselling
2.30–3.00	Tea	
3.00–4.30	Bourn Hall	Sperm cryopreservation in chemotherapy patients. Recent advances in cryo-preservation technology i.e. embryo and ovarian grafts. Counselling cancer patients in relation to fertility therapy
	Discussion	
4.30	Closing Remarks	

Conclusion

This Section concentrated on the process of writing up the report of an enquiry. The way in which findings are presented is very important – not just the language used, but also the structure and the way in which the meaning is conveyed. Conventions for writing reports have been considered and ways of approaching writing have been examined.

The writing process is something which should be going on throughout your enquiry. Writing down ideas, thoughts and questions as they arise is one of the most powerful ways of learning. It is also one of the best ways of finding your own voice.

'After some years it began to happen that I would find myself in the middle of writing a comment and begin to wonder whether it could really be trusted, whether it was really useful. Perhaps I was telling someone about his flowery and wordy diction. His diction was indeed wordy and would be called flowery. But I began to wonder if this was why I was complaining about it. I sometimes found myself suspecting it was something else I couldn't put my finger on that bothered me but floweriness was more available. If I were in a different mood or the paper were in a different place in the stack, perhaps I wouldn't have made the comment I did.'

Elbow, P. (1973) *Writing Without Teachers.* Oxford: Oxford University Press.

Tutor/counsellors and assessors (and anyone else who reads your work) are only human. However hard they may try to be objective, they have good days and bad, as well as particular likes and dislikes.

If you disagree with comments made on drafts of your report, talk about them. Ask for early feedback in a way which means something to you.

References

Cormack, D.F.S. (1986) Writing a research article. *Nurse Education Today* 6:64-68.

Leedy, P. (1989) The review of related literature. In: Leedy, P. *Practical Research: Planning and design* (4th edition) New York: Macmillan.

Strauss, A. and Corbin, J. (1990) *Basics of Qualitative Research. Grounded theory: procedures and techniques.* Newbury Park, Ca.: Sage Publications Inc.

There have been many different voices in this book. By carrying out your own enquiry-based project, you have already added to them in your writing, and by talking to colleagues, friends and other professionals.

Keep enquiring. And keep talking and writing.

'There is of course no absolute distinction between reflection and experience: the most abstract reflection is fed by the memory traces of past experience, and all perceptual experience has a conceptual dimension of interpretation and identification.'

Heron, J. The role of reflection in a cooperative enquiry. In: Boud, D., Keogh, R. and Walker, D. (1985) *Reflection: Turning experience into learning.* London: Kogan Page.

How can your reflection of this unit feed into your experience in the future – and vice versa?